THE 30-DAY CANDIDA CLEANSE

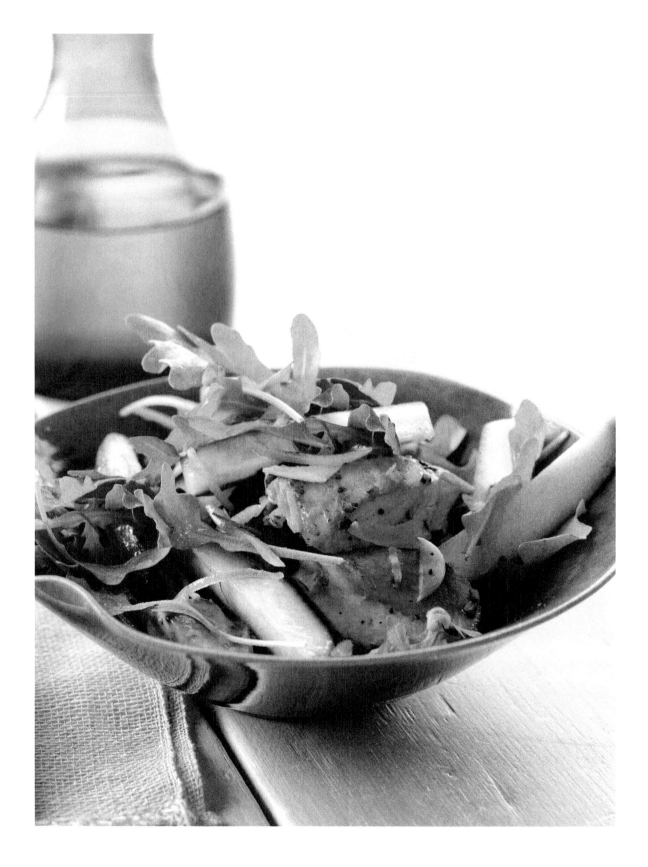

the 30-*day* Candida Cleanse

THE COMPLETE DIET PROGRAM TO
BEAT CANDIDA & RESTORE TOTAL HEALTH

ROCKRIDGE
PRESS

7 Simple Tips to Treat Candida

1 **Eat foods high in iron.** Candida flourishes in a low-oxygen atmosphere so keeping your iron levels up fights the growth of the yeast. Iron helps carry oxygen in the blood, so be sure to include spinach, broccoli, quinoa, lean beef, chicken breast, and pumpkin seeds in your diet.

2 **Let herbs be thy medicine.** Using fresh basil, oregano, cumin, and ginger in your recipes is a great way to enhance taste, and it is also a secret weapon in your candida diet. These herbs, and many others, have antifungal and antiseptic properties, which are powerful candida-overgrowth fighters.

3 **Keep bacteria out.** Leftovers are often a convenient lunch or breakfast the next day, but people with candida can be sensitive to any bacteria on leftover foods, so storage is key. Make sure you chill your food quickly and store it in sealed glass containers with little airspace.

4 **Try it raw.** Eat washed, unpeeled, lightly cooked, or raw vegetables. Vegetable skin contains many important nutrients and cooking can leach away these nutrients.

5 **Go for garlic.** Potent and powerful, garlic is an important food on the candida diet because it is an antifungal and can promote a healthy immune system. Try roasting whole heads of garlic in the oven by cutting off a small section of the top and drizzling the head with olive oil. Bake the garlic in a 350°F oven until it is tender and fragrant. Then squeeze the cloves out of the head and use them in recipes for extra flavor and nutritional benefits.

6 **Pickle it.** Fermented foods are approved candida diet choices, so try making your own pickled vegetables. Look for recipes without sugar and those that use candida diet–approved ingredients.

7 **Enjoy dessert.** Extreme depravation is a sure path to failure. If you are craving a creamy cold dessert, make your own sugar- and dairy-free desserts. If you have an ice cream maker, a combination of almond milk, egg yolks, stevia, and either nuts or candida diet–approved fruit can be a perfect icy end to a healthy dinner.

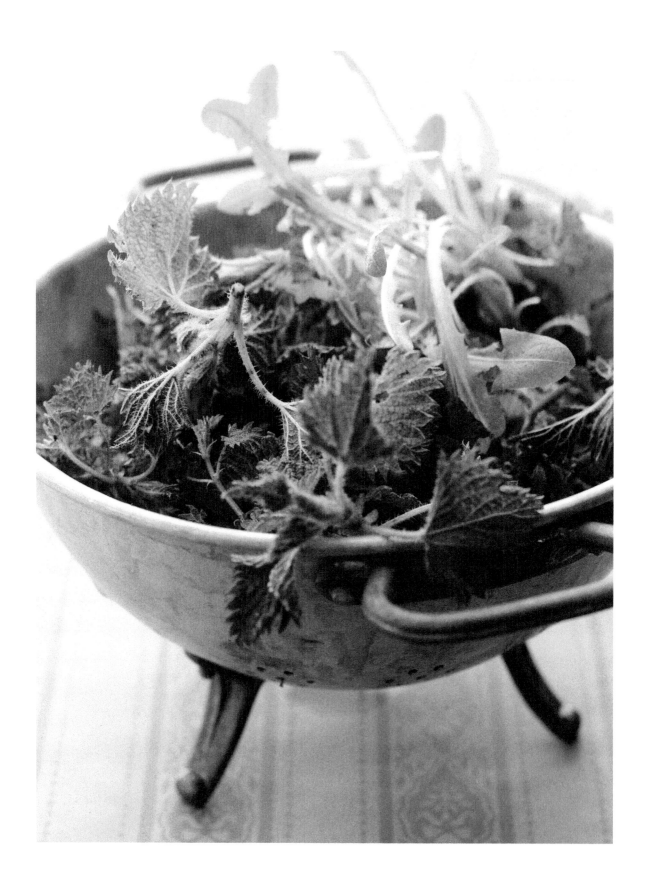

CONTENTS

PART TWO
Candida Diet Recipes

INTRODUCTION

The symptoms of candida overgrowth can be uncomfortable, but they don't have to be a life sentence. Fatigue, acid reflux, headaches, constipation, weight gain, and depression may all sound miserably familiar to you. While your candida sensitivity will not go away over time, you *can* relieve your symptoms and help restore your health by making positive diet choices.

Candida albicans is a common yeast found naturally in the human body. What causes yeast overgrowth isn't completely understood, but it's clear that diet can play a key role in the treatment, control, and possible elimination of candida symptoms. If you suffer from candida sensitivity, gaining control of your life starts with the nutrients you put into your system.

Despite the amount of information published about candida, determining which treatment path will best help combat your candida overgrowth can be a challenge. *The 30-Day Candida Cleanse* helps you navigate the myths and facts surrounding systemic candida overgrowth, provides a simple blueprint for following the candida cleanse and maintenance diet, and offers delicious recipes that will satisfy your appetite.

In chapter 1 you will learn not only what candida is but also the factors that can contribute to yeast overgrowth in your body. A questionnaire will help you understand if the physical symptoms you are experiencing indicate candida sensitivity. Though you may not have received the confirmation and support you want from the medical community thus far, there are tests available to help diagnose a candida sensitivity. Chapter 1 describes these tests along with the traditional and alternative treatments for candida sensitivity, and the limitations of those approaches. Candida treatments are often aimed at specific symptoms rather than at underlying influences, such as the amount of sugar in your diet. Symptoms can be improved with medication, but addressing the influencing conditions (i.e., the foods you eat) can bring about even broader results. And, making changes to your diet is almost always less invasive and has fewer side effects than taking medication.

Chapter 2 explores the relationship between candida sensitivity and diet through a tour of the digestive system and an explanation of how candida affects digestion as well as the other systems in the body. What you eat has a direct impact on whether or not the unhealthy flora, fungi, and bacteria in your body can grow out of control. The candida diet is designed to help you keep this growth in check by outlining the food choices required to combat candida overgrowth. This chapter describes the diet and its two phases—the cleanse phase and the maintenance phase.

When starting a new diet, most people want to know exactly what foods they have to give up to get the results they want. Chapter 3 provides all the approved foods lists for each phase of the diet. You may be surprised, and certainly will feel encouraged, by the variety of foods available to you. Many of your favorite foods may even be found in these lists. Lists of restricted foods are also clearly outlined in this chapter, along with the reasons for excluding these choices from your diet. The pitfalls associated with grocery shopping and eating out while following the candida diet are addressed here, so you can prepare yourself for these activities and ensure you get through them successfully.

After you have a clear understanding of what you can and cannot eat on the candida diet, you may feel a little overwhelmed by the changes required to get your candida overgrowth under control. The thirty-day cleanse and the ninety-day cleanse meal plans walk you through your candida cleanse. A week-long transitional menu supports your move from the cleanse phase into the maintenance stage. Each day's menu plan includes three meals, two substantial snacks, and a dessert, so you will feel satisfied all day long.

The second part of this book is devoted to offering you more than one hundred easy-to-prepare, delicious, and healthy recipes for every meal of the day, including dessert. Yes, there is always room for dessert! The recipes are broken down into cleanse and maintenance categories so you know exactly when to include them in your diet plan.

Remember, this diet is not a short-term quick fix but rather a lifestyle commitment to help keep candida symptoms at bay. The simple diet outlined in this book will soon become second nature to you, and your vibrant good health will be the powerful motivation you need to continue with the plan and a life free of candida symptoms.

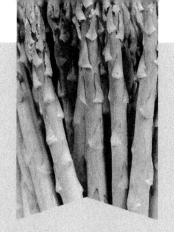

PART I

The Candida Diet

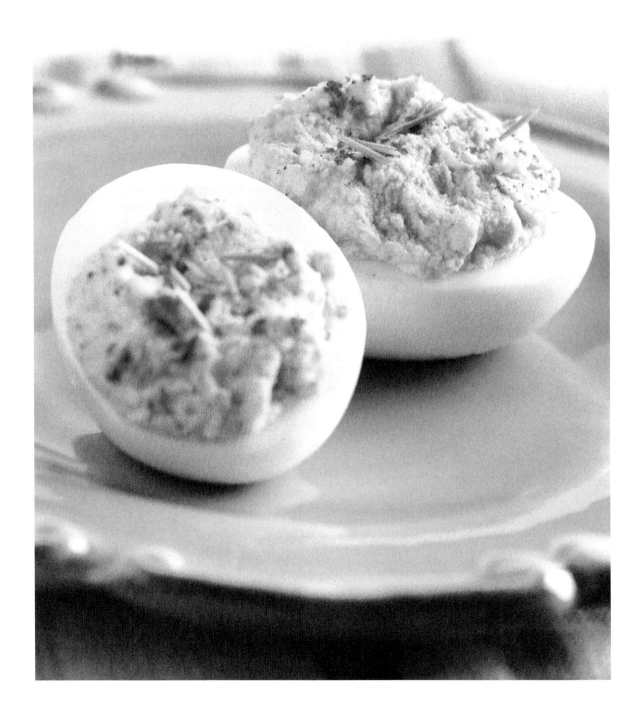

1

What Is Candida?

If you or someone close to you suffers from candida sensitivity, living with the symptoms affects your life every day. The goal of this book is to help you regain control of your life and restore balance to your health. In the chapters that follow, you will find facts and sound reasoning for the candida diet as well as easy, delicious recipes that will help you relieve its symptoms.

Before moving forward, remember a few important points. First, you aren't alone. You or someone close to you suffers, and you may feel failed or betrayed by traditional medicine. You might even hesitate to describe your symptoms to anyone anymore, since you feel crazy trying to tell someone what's wrong. The fact that you are reading this, though, should remind you that there are many others out suffering from the same symptoms. This is a health concern that is more common than you may think.

The Medical Science behind Candida

A full range of ailments can fall under the term "candida," which is more properly called candida sensitivity. Different from candidiasis, candida sensitivity is a controversial condition that many doctors and scientists deny exists but that some medical professionals and scientists acknowledge—and even more laypeople swear that it causes them a range of health problems that disrupt their lives. To understand the controversy, you must first understand the issues.

Candida itself is a fungus, a genus of yeast. *Candida albicans* is the scientific name for most common species of yeast seen in humans. This yeast occurs naturally in all humans because it plays an essential role in digestion and the absorption of nutrients. However, like anything else in your body, the amount of candida matters; normal amounts of candida are slight and concentrated to a small extent in your mouth and to a larger extent in your intestines.

The problem arises when candida is overproduced within your body. When that happens, the resulting condition can reach the level of infection. This is called candidiasis, also known as thrush or a yeast infection. *Andrews' Diseases of the Skin*, a well-respected resource on clinical dermatology, says candidiasis may be referred to as candidosis, moniliasis, and oidiomycosis by your doctor.

When you hear "yeast infection" or "thrush," you may think this isn't a serious health problem. Sometimes that's true, as when the candidiasis is as simple as an infant's thrush, in which the child has a white coating on the tongue, or when the candidiasis manifests as a mild vaginal yeast infection, as most women have experienced. However, don't delude yourself. True candidiasis can also be potentially life-threatening and typically affects people who are severely immunocompromised, such as people with AIDS or cancer, or those who have had an organ transplant or emergency surgery. These more serious infections are called candidemia. The frequency of candida infections is increasing worldwide, and candidemia represents the fourth most common bloodstream infection in the United States, according to a 2005 article in the *Archives of Medical Research*.

It shouldn't surprise you, then, to learn that even less serious health conditions that cause sufferers to be immunocompromised can lead to overproduction of candida and eventual infection. For example, according to the Centers for Disease Control and Prevention, all types of infections, including candidiasis, are more likely to be found in those who suffer from chronic fatigue syndrome (CFS). Since there are at least one million people in the United States who suffer from CFS, to take this example a step further, this group reflects a significant number of people who are grappling with candida overgrowth. This is just one of many ways people can become vulnerable to candida symptoms as a result of being immunocompromised.

Of course, a weakened immune system is not the only factor in candida overgrowth. Because the fungus is associated with digestion and also requires moisture to thrive, it is most likely to overgrow in the mouth, colon, or vagina. Dr. Jack Sobel writes on UpToDate.com that there are multiple risk factors that predict likely vaginal overgrowth. Some of these include the use of douches and other detergents, hormonal fluctuations (including pregnancy, hormone replacement therapy, infertility treatment, and use of birth control pills), use of antibiotics, diabetes mellitus, and even wearing wet swimwear for extended periods of time. These predictive behaviors entail risk because they all disturb the normal vaginal flora, tending to kill off healthy vaginal flora and allow the unhealthy flora to thrive.

Diet may also be linked to rates of candida growth, according to a 1999 study published in the *American Journal of Clinical Nutrition*. The following sections will discuss this in much greater detail, but the general principle is that diets high in simple carbohydrates are friendly for candida overgrowth. This is because carbohydrates, especially simple carbohydrates, break down into glucose (sugar) in your digestive tract very readily. This sugar is what candida lives on. The data so far on whether a high-carbohydrate diet actually does cause candida overgrowth are not conclusive, but proponents of the candida diet base many of their recommendations on the simple idea—not under dispute—that sugars feed yeast.

There are three ways traditional medical doctors usually diagnose a visible candida infection, such as thrush: microscopic examination, culturing, or a combination of both. This is for diagnosis of actual infection, mind you—not candida sensitivity, which we will get to below.

Once your doctor has confirmed candidiasis, the most common treatment is usually an antifungal (also known as antimycotic) drug of some kind. The most frequently prescribed drugs are fluconazole, which is typically taken by mouth, and the topical drugs clotrimazole, ketoconazole, and nystatin. Currently, fluconazole is the most commonly prescribed drug for candidiasis of all types.

However, a 2012 study published in *Obstetrics and Gynecology* found that candida can and does sometimes develop resistance to fluconazole, especially when it must be used repeatedly. This is why some seriously ill patients, such as those with AIDS or candidal blood infections, develop fluconazole resistance and must then pursue alternative candidiasis treatment plans. Usually these consist of intravenous drugs like caspofungin or amphotericin B. Unfortunately, these drugs themselves tend to have serious side effects and cause their users to experience illness and discomfort.

There is a very large group of people—perhaps including you—that experiences many candida-related symptoms but are not diagnosed with candidiasis. In other words, at least according to traditional medical methods, although they have recurring symptoms, the symptoms cannot be proven to be linked to candida. This range of symptoms is what we are referring to as candida sensitivity.

An ongoing debate has raged among most of the traditional medical and scientific communities and the natural or alternative medical community—not to mention people who are not medical practitioners—for years now on this point. Not on how to treat, which drugs are appropriate, or any other details, but on the major question of whether systemic candidiasis, or hypersensitivity to candida, exists at all. Obviously, since you are reading this book, you are probably convinced by your own experience of its existence, but the fact that so many in the medical and scientific communities do not recognize candida sensitivity has perhaps been a serious problem for you.

If so, at least take heart in the fact that you aren't alone. In 1986 Dr. William Crook published his groundbreaking book, *The Yeast Connection*, and since that time candida sensitivity has been a hot topic. The general consensus among sufferers as well as professionals who treat the malady is that candida sensitivity manifests as a series of health problems that occur together as a syndrome: brain fog; fatigue; fingernail and toenail fungus; asthma; depression; skin problems such as rashes, eczema, and psoriasis; irritable bowel syndrome, diarrhea, and other digestive problems; urinary tract problems, sometimes leading to kidney disease; hypoglycemia (low blood sugar); PMS; sexual dysfunction; and muscle pain or even multiple sclerosis.

The main issue with candida sensitivity is thought to be that the candida in the body is not overgrown enough to have caused an infection, so it is technically subclinical, or not localized enough to be detected by a test. However, Crook and others argue that the candida itself has built up enough throughout the system of the sufferer due to poor diet, stress, poor health, a poor immune system, and other factors that the symptoms appear—just not as traditional candidiasis. The belief behind treatment, then, is to eliminate the excess candida, usually with a dietary cleanse, and then to permanently change the sufferer's overall diet in a significant way so that this kind of candida buildup cannot recur.

Certainly, the modern diet in the United States would support candida overgrowth. Rife with convenience foods and other overprocessed foods heavy with simple carbohydrates and sugars, the standard American diet is exactly what candida thrives on. In his original anti-candida manifesto, Crook called for eating a diet focused on fresh foods. He also insisted that foods high in yeast and sugars must be avoided, along with fermented foods (which are themselves typically sugary and yeasty) such as vinegar and alcohol.

Since Crook's book was published in 1986, many people have tried changing their health by changing their diets. Many have been living with candida sensitivity with varying degrees of success, and with varying levels of medical treatment. The most modern approach to candida sensitivity is truly the much easier, healthier, and more effective means of seeking balance for your body and managing your symptoms together with your doctor.

Questionnaire: Do You Have Candida Sensitivity?

If you are still not sure about whether candida sensitivity is your problem, go over this list of questions carefully. They concern common signs of candida sensitivity and a buildup of candida in the body. If you answer yes to many of the questions here, you may have candida sensitivity.

Do You Get Frequent Fungal Infections of the Skin and Nails?

Some examples of this include athlete's foot, fungal infections on the skin under the breasts or in the armpit creases, or toenail fungus that turns your toenails very thick and yellow. Fungal skin and nail infections are, unfortunately, very common for those with candida sensitivity and, according to the National Institutes of Health, are linked to the presence of excessive *Candida albicans* in the body.

As with other symptoms you experience with candida sensitivity, these fungal skin and nail infections are a sign of more significant problems associated with a weakened immune system, along with poor blood circulation and, at times, a lack of oxygen in the blood. But be careful: It is crucial to use caution while you check for these skin infections, because other skin problems, such as eczema and psoriasis, look very similar and also occur frequently in those who suffer from candida sensitivity. These problems can be serious, so get medical help when you aren't sure what you're looking at.

Do You Suffer from Exhaustion, Frequent Feelings of Being Worn Out, Chronic Fatigue, or Fibromyalgia?

More than one million Americans experience some form of extreme fatigue, according to the Centers for Disease Control and Prevention (CDC). In fact, fatigue is one of the most common ailments in the United States for which people seek help, and one of the most common questions that doctors and other health professionals hear concerning fatigue is, "How do I know if this is really chronic fatigue or if I'm just feeling worn out?" This question becomes even more difficult to answer given that chronic fatigue symptoms are very difficult for traditional medicine to definitively diagnose.

Like candida sensitivity, chronic fatigue lends itself to treatment with natural medicine, and in fact is often a component of the overall candida syndrome. Crook and some other doctors believe candida buildup in the body, along with eating foods that contain too much yeast, sugar, and other chemicals that can trigger sensitivities in certain people, are the primary dietary causes of fatigue for Americans.

Do You Experience Ongoing Digestive Problems Such As Bloating, Constipation, Diarrhea, Spastic Colon, Irritable Bowel Syndrome, or Gas?

A host of digestive problems may be associated with candida sensitivity and systemic buildup of candida. Some of them can be quite serious: Significant fungal colonization

WHAT IS CHRONIC FATIGUE SYNDROME?

According to the CDC, chronic fatigue syndrome (CFS) is a disorder that causes extreme fatigue that limits your ability to function in your everyday activities. This fatigue is not the kind of tired feeling that goes away after you rest. The key way to distinguish CFS from just being tired is a feeling of severe fatigue that lasts six months or more, along with at least four of these other symptoms:

- Joint pain in several areas
- Persistent muscle pain
- Physical activity causes you to feel sickness or pain for more than twenty-four hours afterward
- Recurrent headaches

- Significant memory problems
- Sleep problems
- Sore throat without apparent cause
- Tender lymph nodes

There are no tests for CFS; it is a diagnosis made by excluding all other possibilities. It occurs most often in women in their forties and fifties. Lifestyle changes and coping techniques are at the heart of CFS treatment, because there is no cure at this time.

of the colon, most often with candida, may influence the activation of ulcerative colitis, according to researchers at Jagiellonian University in Poland. Candida has also been found proliferating in the gut of people with irritable bowel syndrome (IBS).

When candida buildup goes unchecked, every piece of food you eat ferments in your system instead of simply getting digested. The buildup and resulting fermenting mess can penetrate the lining of the intestines. The entire gut or digestive system becomes increasingly inflamed by this cycle. This level of candida buildup is usually referred to as leaky gut, because it can cause breaches in the walls of the gut. This triggers an immune response in the bloodstream—and the next level of trouble.

Do You Have an Autoimmune Disease Such As Hashimoto's Thyroiditis, Rheumatoid Arthritis, Ulcerative Colitis, Lupus, Psoriasis, Scleroderma, or Multiple Sclerosis?

Hashimoto's thyroiditis, rheumatoid arthritis, ulcerative colitis, lupus, psoriasis, scleroderma, multiple sclerosis, and similar diseases may be linked to leaky gut. Most naturopaths believe that the large proteins circulating in the body as the result of leaky gut syndrome can result in food sensitivities and even allergies, as these get into the bloodstream and trigger inflammation and an immune response. This means the immune system mounts a response to fight them. When *Candida albicans* is part of this invasion, the immune system "remembers" the candida when it sees the fungus in the future.

This is the same way vaccinations work: An immune response is triggered so that your immune system can "remember" the disease and form antibodies that will fight it in the future. So why is this kind of exposure a good thing when it comes to vaccinations but a bad thing when it comes to candida? Because the immune system is then primed to react to all foods containing yeast and fungi: It cannot distinguish an attack from a piece of white bread.

Candida sensitivity has been linked to celiac disease, and may have an important connection to autoimmune disorders, according to the Denver Naturopath Clinic. A study published in a 2012 issue of *Nature* showed that some fungi activate the immune cells involved in the development of autoimmune illnesses, while other convey an anti-inflammatory function. The researchers concluded that the composition of microflora in our bodies plays a decisive role in the development of some chronic illnesses.

Do You Have Difficulty Concentrating, Poor Memory, Lack of Focus, ADD, ADHD, and/or Brain Fog?

If you have any of these concentration problems, you may be experiencing one of the most common symptom clusters of candida sensitivity. Brain fog or difficulty concentrating was originally associated with multiple sclerosis, states WebMD, and is one of the more distressing symptoms of that disease (aside from pain). Brain fog is also one of the more common candida-related mental complaints. There is no formal way to recognize something like brain fog—unlike a formal diagnosis of dementia, for example. Instead, the sufferer simple feels "off," cannot concentrate, and reports that he or she lacks clarity. While this is subjective and difficult to diagnose, the reports among those who suffer from candida sensitivity are also fairly consistent.

Whenever candida yeast either grows or dies, acetaldehydes are released. These chemicals are the product of yeast fermentation, and are what causes a hangover after too much drinking. A steady stream of them in the body can interfere with proper brain function.

This is why natural practitioners sometimes link ADD or ADHD to candida. This, they say, is why food allergies as well as candida buildup are sometimes a problem for ADD or ADHD sufferers (and vice versa). There is currently no definitive evidence proving a link between candida and ADHD, but sufferers who have changed their diet have reported improvement, and, according to the National Resource Center on ADHD, a combination of antifungal drugs and a candida diet are commonly prescribed as complementary and alternative treatments for ADHD.

Do You Have a Skin Disease Such As Eczema, Psoriasis, Hives, or Rashes?

Skin diseases like eczema, psoriasis, hives, and certain other rashes are considered autoimmune conditions. These also may be a sign of candida sensitivity and buildup in the body. Candida particles produce a byproduct that can be toxic in large amounts. A buildup of candida causes that byproduct to spread throughout the body, causing an overreaction from your immune system that can result in these skin problems. Once again, the immune system cannot distinguish between candida and real threats to the body.

The scaly, itchy skin that comes with most of these conditions is usually treated with anti-inflammatory and immunosuppressant drugs, but this actually makes candida buildup worse. That's because these drugs also kill off the beneficial flora in your body, allowing candida to proliferate with less competition. And, as we have already discussed, overgrowth of detrimental bacteria has been shown to have a link to autoimmune illnesses.

Do You Suffer from Irritability, Mood Swings, Anxiety, or Depression?

Irritability, mood swings, anxiety, and depression unrelated to life events have all been linked anecdotally with candida sensitivity and are also among the most frightening of the symptoms. At first you might doubt that psychological symptoms could be a part of candida sensitivity, but when you think it through, it shouldn't be surprising to you that your brain is sensitive to mycotoxins, the toxic byproducts of candida.

Candida sensitivity and buildup can cause many psychological and psychiatric symptoms—if for no other reason than sufferers find themselves sad and frustrated at being persistently ill. The most common symptoms are anxiety and depression. However, reported symptoms may also include irritability, angry outbursts, obsessive-compulsive activities, mood swings, paranoia, panic attacks, serious crying spells, personality changes, and, at times, even behavior that may be characterized as schizophrenic, according to Dr. Crook. (It is important to be under the care of a mental health professional if you experience serious mental health symptoms.)

WHEN IS IT TIME TO SEEK PROFESSIONAL HELP FOR DEPRESSION?

There's no doubt that lifestyle changes, including a healthy diet and exercise, can affect your mood in important ways. However, there are times when depression and other mental health issues become so serious that it is crucial to seek out professional help. Here are some factors to consider when you're thinking about whether you can manage your depression yourself with some lifestyle changes, or if you need to seek the help of a professional. According to the National Institutes of Health:

- A major depressive disorder causes you severe trouble with your ability to eat, sleep, study or work, and generally enjoy your life.
- Psychotic depression is characterized by symptoms of severe depression plus some disturbing false beliefs or break with reality, such as delusions or hallucinations.
- Postpartum depression versus the "baby blues" will feel overwhelming and will last longer than several months after giving birth. It will also interfere with your ability to complete even the most basic tasks.
- Seasonal affective disorder is caused by lack of natural sunlight in winter months, and typically appears in that season.

If you have one or more of these signs, talk to a mental health professional.

Do You Suffer from Frequent Vaginal Infections, Urinary Tract Infections, Rectal Itching, or Vaginal Itching?

These kinds of infections are associated with candida buildup because the vagina, penis, and colon are common areas for candida, and an imbalance of healthy flora causes these kinds of problems. Urinary tract infections (UTIs) are statistically most often a result of bacterial infection, but as scientists report in the *Review of Infectious Diseases*, those that are caused by candida tend to arise from genital candida overgrowth.

Similarly, if you experience frequent rectal itching or vaginal itching, it may be a result of candida buildup. The itching may or may not indicate infection, of course. Some symptoms of vaginal candidiasis defined by the Centers for Disease Control and Prevention include itching, redness of the vulva, pain while urinating, a thick white vaginal discharge that looks somewhat like cottage cheese and may smell yeasty, and occasionally, whitish patches on the skin of the vulva. Generally, discharge associated with candidiasis isn't foul-smelling. (Being immunocompromised can make you more susceptible to other kinds of infections, and those may present a foul-smelling discharge.) Typically, the presence of localized candida causes itching—most commonly in the area of the vagina or penis.

Do You Suffer from Severe Seasonal Allergies, Itchy Ears, or Chronic Sinusitis?

If you have severe seasonal allergies, itchy ears, or chronic sinusitis, this may be another indicator of candida sensitivity, according to a French study published in *Allergie et Immunologie (Paris)*. As we have already discussed, candida cells can trigger an overreaction from your immune system. This causes inflammation and a severe response from certain specialized immune cells. This immune response can become an allergy. Over time, as your body fights your allergic symptoms, the effort causes your adrenal glands to work too hard. This can in turn lead to adrenal fatigue or non-Addison's hypoadrenia—a collection of symptoms that appear when the adrenal glands function below the necessary level. Healthy adrenal glands regulate many functions in the body, and adrenal disorders can affect many systems.

Do You Feel Strong Cravings for Sugars and Refined Carbohydrates?

If you feel strong or even out-of-control cravings for sugars and refined carbohydrates, you may be suffering from candida sensitivity, according to the website Natural News. As if the rest of it wasn't bad enough, as you try to put yourself back on track, candida sensitivity can even make you feel at war with yourself because you crave exactly what you shouldn't be eating. Candida ferments sugars into alcohol, which destabilizes your blood sugar level. The candida is simply surviving, but the result is that you feel intense and immediate cravings for more and more simple carbohydrates and sugar.

How Your Doctor's Treatments Work with the Candida Diet

Since there is so much disagreement in the medical community about the very existence of candida sensitivity, is there a way to be in harmony with your doctor about your treatment? What options can you expect your doctor to present to you? And first, how can you be tested for candida sensitivity or buildup?

While most doctors will certainly test for candidiasis if they believe such testing is indicated, many traditional medical doctors don't believe in candida sensitivity. Therefore, how to test for it isn't simple. However, there are some recommended approaches from the experts.

Many practitioners of alternative medicine believe that stool testing is a good way to test for candida sensitivity. The experts affiliated with the website WholeApproach say that extended stool testing can show which treatment will work for you, because stool testing can discern the species of yeast that is present. There is also a urine-based test for candida buildup. The Organix Dysbiosis urine test looks for a candida waste product, D-arabinitol. An elevated result indicates a possible buildup of candida, and it should also indicate whether the buildup is in your upper digestive tract or your small intestine. There are also blood tests available that can check for high levels of candida antibodies: IgG, IgA, and IgM antibodies may indicate candida buildup. These are less sensitive than both the stool and urine tests and present with many false negatives compared to both the other tests.

If you determine that you have a candida buildup, you will face another potential problem: Traditional medical treatments may make it worse. Treatments for candidiasis generally include antifungal drugs or antimycotics, and these are the same treatments that you will probably receive for candida buildup. The most commonly prescribed drugs are fluconazole (usually taken orally) and the topical drugs clotrimazole, ketoconazole, and nystatin. However, candida can develop resistance to fluconazole, according to a 1995 study published in *Antimicrobial Agents and Chemotherapy*. The problem is that the drugs used in fluconazole-resistant patients, such as intravenous drugs like caspofungin or amphotericin B, can have serious side effects.

If you are diagnosed with chronic fatigue syndrome, you will likely be told that currently there is no truly effective treatment for problem. If you are diagnosed with any of the digestive disorders caused by candida sensitivity, you will probably be given natural fiber treatments. While the fiber does not damage your body, it is ineffective against the candida buildup and can actually increase bloating and gas.

Additionally, as the candida buildup worsens, the fermentation in your gut does too. The inflammation in your gut also worsens and candida is more and more likely to enter your bloodstream. This leads to more immune system overreactions, and more trouble with immunosuppressive diseases and allergies. Your doctor may give you anti-inflammatories and immunosuppressant drugs as these symptoms continue, but this can actually help the candida build up even more as the natural flora that would normally compete with it are killed off by the drugs.

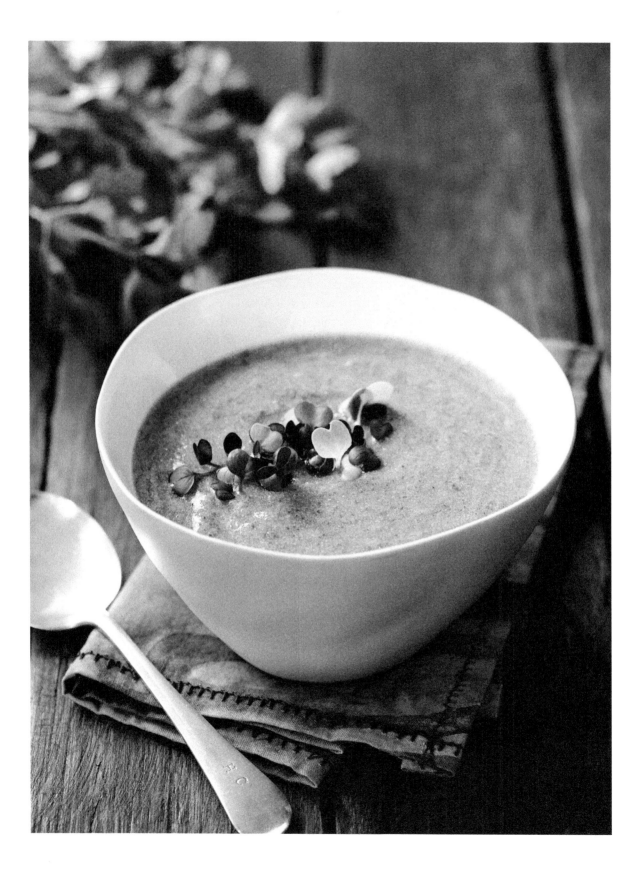

2

Candida and Food

There is almost nothing as basic or intimate to our lives as the food we eat, so it is no wonder that a candida sensitivity problem can feel so overwhelming. There is simply no question that if candida buildup and sensitivity are causing you health problems, there is a connection to the food you eat. This may make you feel as if the problem is too much for anyone to control. However, there is an alternate view: The fact that candida sensitivity and diet are so interconnected means you can take control of your symptoms.

When you look at the world we live in and imagine any one creature somehow multiplying until it is out of control, you realize that this kind of imbalance poses a major problem to the rest of the system. A plague of locusts, for example, would destroy crops at a minimum, causing a chain reaction affecting species all over the globe. Thinking of your body as an ecosystem, you can see candida buildup starting a chain reaction throughout your body. The first impact is probably on your digestive system or genital area, but eventually the rest of the system will suffer. For a better understanding of the intimate connection between food and candida, let's take a closer look.

The Digestive System and How It Relates to Candida

Digestion is breaking down food and extracting what is needed to keep the body healthy, while eliminating what is unneeded or unhealthy. To function properly, the digestive system, or gastrointestinal (GI) tract, requires many different organs to work together in the right way as part of a complex process. The GI tract itself functions as a kind of membrane, a tube letting only the useful portions of the food into the body and rejecting the rest. A GI tract that is functioning well is able to be selective without much trouble.

In digestion there are four basic steps: processing, absorption, assimilation, and elimination. When your mouth chews and salivates and your stomach further breaks down the food you eat, your system is processing the food and readying it for absorption. The absorption step begins in earnest in the small intestine, where the lion's share of nutrients cross over into the bloodstream. Next, the nutrients are assimilated into the body's cells. And finally, the rejected portions of food go on to the large intestine and then the colon, from which they are eliminated.

Your body needs a great deal of energy to get the work of digestion done. Your GI tract demands a relatively large blood supply—one-third of your overall blood supply, in fact, according to *Connections*, a publication of Women's International Pharmacy. When your digestive system is hard at work, your body diverts even more blood than usual to your GI tract (which is why you might feel cold after a large meal as blood rushes from your periphery to aid in the digestion of your food).

Healthy digestion requires healthy flora, as scientists explain in a 2003 study published in the *Lancet*. Your stomach, intestines, and colon contain more than four hundred species of bacteria, almost all of them beneficial to your digestive process. Most adults have between five and eight pounds of these bacteria, which live mainly in the colon. They are so important to healthy digestion because they ferment the food we eat, producing nutrients, and they also feed the cells of the GI tract with short-chain fatty acids that they produce. Your GI tract cannot function without these bacteria.

Candida albicans is another part of your healthy GI tract. Normal conditions within the GI tract maintain a balance that keeps your level of candida harmless. However, when your system is out of balance (for whatever reason), you can experience a buildup of candida. This is where the problems start.

In general, replacing the friendly bacteria in the GI tract with any unfriendly bacteria, fungus, or parasites, including candida, causes inflammation, according to Medical News Today. This affects surrounding cells and organs, and the inflammation spreads. However, candida buildup also has its own specific problems that compound the issue.

Candida can disrupt normal hormone function in your body because it binds with estrogen, preventing it from being used properly by the body and leading to a buildup of progesterone—the hormone that creates a balance to estrogen levels. A study published in *Clinical and Experimental Immunology* found that the production of antibodies to candida is influenced by the naturally occurring fluctuations in hormones during a woman's menstrual cycle. This helps explain why, in women, candida overgrowth can fluctuate. But it's important to remember that both men and women need estrogen, and that its production is inhibited by candida overgrowth.

As already discussed, the buildup of candida in the intestines also causes a wide variety of chronic digestive problems, including bloating, diarrhea, acid reflux, and inflammation. Other symptoms include headaches, fatigue, muscle aches and spasms, chronic sinusitis, and flu-like symptoms. Candida buildup is also often associated with diseases that affect women, such as endometriosis, imbalance of hormones, vaginitis, pain in the breasts, and chronic trouble with vaginal discharge, vaginal yeast infections, urinary tract infections, and premenstrual syndrome.

How Diet and Candida Are Related

Under normal circumstances, the healthy bacteria in your body maintain balanced levels of candida and other potentially dangerous flora in the GI tract. However, modern life features so many factors that allow candida levels to spiral out of control.

A diet laden with simple, processed, or refined carbohydrates causes candida to overgrow, according to the website Smart Nutrition. As the Harvard School of Public Health Nutrition Source explains, that's because sugars and simple carbohydrates are yeast fuel—end of story. This kind of diet also causes blood sugar levels to spike and plummet. Blood sugar comes from the foods you eat and from energy stored in your body. When your blood sugar level drops, your body either takes in more or uses up its stores. When blood sugar spikes, your body secretes insulin that enables the cells to metabolize glucose. This isn't a problem in and of itself; clearly, your body needs energy. However, diets too high in sugars and processed carbohydrates—including the typical modern American diet—cause intense, cyclic cravings for even more simple carbohydrates and sugar.

The result is a terrible, self-perpetuating cycle. You've been there! You know what happens. Eventually you give in. This is especially true when you are busy or stressed and you are unprepared. At the last minute when you feel starved, your cravings are the strongest, even though you know logically that you are not actually starving. This strong craving leads you to choose more sugary, simple carbohydrates and highly processed foods.

Certainly, most people know that eating this way can make them gain weight, and they also know that perhaps this sort of eating makes them feel not quite their best. But the idea that a white-bread and high-sugar diet can cause serious, chronic health problems is difficult for many people to accept. Remember, American culture has historically equated family and celebrations with things like cake, ice cream, candy, hot dogs, hamburgers, and French fries.

Getting Ready for the Candida Diet

Does the idea of completely overhauling your diet seem intimidating? If it does, consider this: You have almost certainly seen a medical doctor at some point about some of your health problems, without any success. You've felt compelled to research the issue on your own, and even though you've discovered numerous facts, you haven't yet found anything that has restored your health. The real question now is: What do you have to lose?

On the candida diet, you change the foods you eat every day, for a set period of time. You'll be doing so to restore your health. When you consider that diet change may be all you need to feel well again, why would you stop yourself?

According to candida diet expert Lisa Richards, author of *The Candida Diet*, there are two basic steps in the candida sensitivity cleanse and diet. (Like those at LiveStrong.com, some see the gradual reintroduction of foods into your diet as its own step; those who do say that there are three steps.) First, you cleanse your body of the candida buildup. Next, you transition into the long-term maintenance diet that will help you avoid future buildups. You transition into that maintenance step only when your body is ready; you are waiting for your health to improve in such a significant way that the change is obvious. As your body goes through this change and the candida dies off, you will feel different. The typical cleanse takes about fourteen days (and sometimes even fewer, depending on how quickly your symptoms are alleviated, says Richards). You can do anything for fourteen days! And once you've developed your new eating habits, if you need to extend your cleanse, it'll be easier than you think.

Changing your diet is never easy or simple. Eliminating all the foods that feed candida can be a real challenge. The fact is, you will have to rethink a major part of your life: eating. When people quit smoking, they often have to rethink social activities, alcohol consumption, and other activities and habits that have become entangled with smoking for them, psychologically and physically. When it comes to candida, you will need to transform the way you look at food, especially sugar, yeast, and carbohydrates.

Even without a clinical diagnosis of candidiasis, fighting candida buildup using diet alone can take up to six months, so be aware of this commitment as you begin. Because this process can be so challenging and time consuming, many people do seek out a doctor's advice while they rid their bodies of candida buildup and use antifungal medications as they change their diets. There are alternatives, if either your current diagnosis does not warrant this kind of prescription or if you simply want to avoid taking drugs.

A caprylic acid supplement is one option to try, according to Richards. Caprylic acid supplements are derived from coconut oil, and this natural antifungal substance can also be found naturally in palm oil, human milk, and cow's milk. In 2012, the FDA indicated that the supplement was safe, although it has not approved it for killing candida, which is its most common use.

Probiotic supplements are another great option to try in your fight against candida buildup. They restore the healthy flora balance in your intestines by replenishing the good bacteria, and can help keep candida under control by inhibiting its growth. Probiotics come in different strengths or concentrations, with anything from one billion to one hundred billion or more bacteria per dose, according to the Harvard Health Publications. Although there is no danger in taking probiotics, it is advisable to start conservatively with your dose and later increase the dosage as your body adjusts.

Some probiotic supplements contain only one kind of bacteria, and others contain more than a dozen. Remember that your probiotic should contain a mix of strains, and include the ones that are most potent. These include *Bifidobacteria bifidus* and *Lactobacillus acidophilus*. *Lactobacillus acidophilus* DDS-1 is a more potent strain, and is even better. Although some probiotics also contain prebiotics, which are ostensibly included to assist the probiotics, these are not actually needed, so avoid paying extra for these, suggests *Health Magazine*.

Oil of oregano is another option some people use to fight candida buildup. Unfortunately, oil of oregano can also kill some varieties of beneficial bacteria, states the Adëeva website, and since any candida buildup is itself a systemic imbalance, this option is not ideal. Instead, stick to yeast-specific treatments such as any antifungals your doctor prescribes, and supplements such as caprylic acid and probiotics.

In the initial stage of your candida diet, as you fight the buildup of candida in your system, you will make major changes. You will remove all sugars, breads, yeasts, simple carbohydrates, grains, fruits, most dairy, many vegetables, and almost all processed foods from your diet. Before you throw this book away, wait! This sounds intimidating, to be sure. However, the tips and recipes in this cookbook will make it possible for you to do it. And as you press on, at almost every stage of your process, you will discover that you feel even better than you expected. In fact, at times you may not believe just how different and wonderful your body feels.

Keep track of your progress using this book and your own sense of your body and your health, and you will know when it is time to transition out of the initial cleanse stage of the diet, which is much more restrictive, and move on to the maintenance stage, which is far easier to follow. During the maintenance stage, you can add more vegetables and some fruit back into your diet. You'll feel much more at ease with the candida diet as a whole, and you'll see yourself making dietary choices much more easily. You may even lose weight without trying.

There is one relatively minor side effect to starting this diet that you should be aware of, Richards warns: The Herxheimer reaction, named for the Austrian dermatologist who discovered it, refers to the way your symptoms may appear to worsen for a day or two before they get better. This is actually a sign that the diet is working. The Herxheimer reaction occurs in this case because as large amounts of candida die off, they release toxins. This might cause you to experience chills, fatigue, fever, headache, muscle pain, or skin breakouts. If you do, they will last for only a few days at most, and it is just as likely that you won't experience any of these side effects at all. Understandably, the Herxheimer reaction can be a challenging time. It is crucial to remember that this is a sign of your body healing and an indicator of the balance that is gradually returning to your system.

A Candida Diet Overview

As challenging as the candida diet can seem at first, once you get into the swing of things it is very easy to follow. Here are some basic tips to keep in mind that can guide you to success.

Avoid sweets. As you know, all sugars, even natural ones such as honey and those that occur in fruit, feed candida. You may not realize, however, that almost all artificial sweeteners are also off the list. That leaves stevia, a natural sweetener (more about this in chapter 3). So all foods and beverages that are sweet are to be avoided, unless you've

HOW MUCH WATER IS ENOUGH?

You have probably heard that you should drink eight eight-ounce glasses of water each day, but is that correct? Actually, the answer varies, based on your activity level, size, and health, and the humidity and temperature where you live. So what should you aim for? According to the Institute of Medicine of the National Academies, about 100 ounces (about 3 liters) of liquids, total, in a day works for the average man, while around 75 ounces (about 2.2 liters) of liquids, total, in a day works for the average woman.

sweetened them yourself with nothing but stevia. Their sweetness always comes from something, and that something almost always feeds candida.

Eat bitter and sour foods. Although you may have avoided them in the past, bitter and sour foods are great for you. Some examples of bitter and sour foods include pure, unsweetened aloe vera juice with no additives, dandelion greens and roots, endive, lemon juice, mustard greens, radicchio, radishes, spinach, and other leafy greens. These foods fight your cravings for sweets because they contain enzymes that help your body digest your food. They also improve renal function. By counteracting your cravings for sweets with these healthy bitter and sour foods, you will gradually overcome your cravings, encourages Dr. Prem Jagyasi on his website.

Avoid alcohol. Let's face it; alcohol isn't great for you anyway. But the real reason candida sufferers need to avoid it is that it is instant fuel for candida. Fermented beverages such as beer already contain yeast. And all alcohol converts to sugar right away in your bloodstream, according to MedicineNet.com.

Drink a lot of water. Drinking water is all good for your body; most of us are dehydrated anyway. When you are on the candida diet, especially the initial stage while fighting candida buildup, you are flushing your digestive system. You need to eliminate toxins from your body and cleanse your renal system. And, of course, most other beverages are not really an option on the diet.

Avoid fermented foods. Fermented foods cause gut fermentation—already a problem if you have candida buildup. The few exceptions are fermented foods with probiotic qualities: yogurt, sauerkraut, kefir (a fermented milk beverage), kimchi, and apple cider vinegar. Make sure to buy the raw, all-natural, unpasteurized, or active culture forms of these foods, so their probiotic qualities have not been processed out. Or better yet, make them yourself.

Make stress reduction a priority. This is not strictly diet-related, but it is important to the candida diet. We now know that the intensity of any allergic reaction can be heightened by stress, and candida buildup and sensitivity are seriously affected by the physical changes that accompany stress.

Limit your consumption of antibiotics, oral contraceptives, and other hormones as much as possible. If you must take antibiotics or hormones, also take a good probiotic supplement. (See page 19 for suggestions about probiotics.)

Make your food from scratch whenever possible. When you make it yourself in your own kitchen, you know exactly what's in your food and in what proportions. When you prepare your food yourself using only candida-safe ingredients, you eliminate the risk and guesswork that may otherwise plague your food choices.

Order simple dishes at restaurants. When you do eat out, opt for simple entrées, and ask questions. Dishes with complicated sauces, preparations involving many steps, and rich sides are almost guaranteed to be trouble when you're on the candida diet. You must be able to identify everything on your plate, and you must also know how it is prepared. Ask questions! Don't be afraid to ask a server what is in something. These days, people who are in the business of making and serving food are, by necessity, very aware of food allergies and sensitivities. They want you to know if you are exposing yourself to something you shouldn't eat.

If you are in doubt about any food, avoid it. While you may sometimes be tempted to take a chance, especially if you feel bored with your food, don't! Instead, find a new, exciting recipe to try. If you aren't completely certain whether an ingredient is on your safe list, avoid it. Give it time; after you stick to this rule for a while, the way you feel—your returning health—will make you glad you did.

Criticisms of the Candida Diet

Many medical doctors and scientists do not believe candida sensitivity or candida buildup are actual health problems. They do not believe that there is any such syndrome, and point to the fact that the existence of the syndrome or the efficacy of the diet have never been tested in scientific studies. Candidiasis, they say, is the only health problem proven to be caused by candida. Typically, naturopaths, holistic and alternative medicine practitioners, and some nutrition experts are the ones recommending the candida diet to improve a variety of health problems. They say nutrition is an often-overlooked tool in the health care arsenal, and that positive results for many people speak for themselves. They also say that just because something has not been formally studied does not mean it doesn't work. You need to have all the facts, so here are some summaries of these viewpoints so you may draw your own conclusions.

It is the position of the American Academy of Allergy, Asthma, and Immunology (AAAAI) that the idea of a hypersensitivity to candida is unproven. The AAAAI position statement on this topic finds the concept of candida sensitivity problematic and expresses concern about the syndrome. They feel that the elements of the syndrome are too broad, leading them to potentially apply to almost anyone. They state that the concept of candida sensitivity syndrome is speculative and unproven. And they feel that belief in the syndrome may be causing some people to misuse or overuse antifungal drugs.

If this last argument is true, the concern is that this pattern could lead to the creation of fungi that are resistant to drugs and possible side effects from overuse in people. Thus far, no drug-resistant fungi have been described in the literature, however, and side effects related to antifungal drug overuse are reportedly very rare. In any event, no controlled trials to study these issues have been conducted, according to the website Quackwatch.

The FDA has taken issue with certain candida sensitivity treatments. It is illegal in the United States to sell any product specifically for the prevention or treatment of a disease without FDA approval. Anything sold for those purposes, even natural supplements or food, is considered to be a drug, even if the seller doesn't call it that. Both individual doctors and the company Nature's Way were penalized by the FDA for either diagnosing the syndrome or selling candida "cures." According to the FTC news release posted on the website Casewatch, in the 1980s, Nature's Way sold natural supplements labeled as cures for candidiasis, or actual yeast infections. The company paid a $30,000 settlement to the National Institutes of Health, based on their admission of wrongdoing, after the FDA's fraud branch investigated this practice in 1989. They also stopped marketing the product as a yeast infection cure. According to Quackwatch, two doctors in New Jersey were also barred by the FDA from diagnosing "candida overgrowth syndrome," citing the fact that the syndrome had not been generally recognized or accepted in the medical community.

There are also some criticisms of the candida diet itself. Most of these are rooted in the argument that the diet is too restrictive. Especially in the initial stage designed to eliminate candida buildup, many otherwise very healthy foods are eliminated from the diet, and carbohydrate consumption is severely limited. The criticism is that many of the symptoms attributed to candida sensitivity, such as brain fog, depression, fatigue, inability to concentrate, and mood swings, might actually be exacerbated by such as restricted diet—if not caused by it.

The Mayo Clinic is skeptical about the existence of candida sensitivity syndrome and the diet's ability to cure any health problem. Their position is that when you eliminate sugar, white flour, and processed foods from your diet, you are bound to feel better. On the candida diet, you cut out high-calorie foods with low nutritional value and replace them with high-quality, healthy foods. In other words, you simply improve your diet, which is unrelated to candida buildup. The takeaway for the Mayo Clinic is that eating a healthy diet as a matter of course will eventually cause you to feel better, have more energy, and experience better overall health. Therefore, the fact that the diet benefits your health isn't proof of any problem with candida per se; instead, it is proof that good nutrition benefits your health.

We'll speak to these criticisms point by point, starting with the AAAAI position statement. It is a fact that the syndrome itself has not been proven within the scientific community, that some studies have suggested it does not exist, and that there have been no clinical trials proving the efficacy of the candida diet. The most serious complaint of the AAAAI has to do with prescription drug overuse, and this is unrelated to the actual diet. It is worth noting that there is never a justification for using a prescription drug without cause, and the candida diet certainly doesn't advocate this. Doctors and naturopaths who recommend the diet agree that you must be under the care of a medical doctor if you are taking any antifungal drugs, and that you must avoid taking unnecessary drugs. However, there is no denying the fact that people have their own experiences. Without clinical trials, anecdotal evidence is all we have. Many, many people have found that after years of suffering, this change in their diet finally worked for them.

The FDA issues are also worth considering, but again, they are not related to the actual diet. The FDA can and should watch the actions of businesses and professionals closely as part of its mandate. But individuals seeking to improve their health with their dietary choices isn't really in the same arena as FDA labeling on products marketed as medications.

Of all the criticisms, the restrictiveness of the diet is probably the most important to consider. Any time you follow a diet with a lot of limitations, no matter what your motivation, it is absolutely critical to carefully monitor your body's response. This is not just about watching for symptoms of candida, or of the Herxheimer reaction, but for all the ways your body is responding to the diet change. If your new diet is causing you serious difficulty—more than you can handle—you should change your approach.

Every person is different, and each person's dietary needs are unique. Paying attention to your body is your single best tool in adjusting your intake appropriately. You may need to eat more, or less, or eat a little differently.

Given that this diet provides you with three full meals, two satisfying snacks, and one dessert every day, you should never be hungry (except right before it's time to eat). If you find yourself wanting to eat more, do it; just choose the from your Foods to Enjoy list. Finally, and most important, if your health gets worse in any way, stop the diet at once and seek medical attention as needed.

Even if the Mayo Clinic is right about candida sensitivity, they are also right that when you change your diet this way, you are going to experience better health. Far from being a reason to reject the diet, this is another powerful reason to try this method of fighting your candida sensitivity symptoms. You already know you will feel better. So why not?

Q&A: Is the Candida Diet Right for You?

No matter how good or effective it is, no single diet is right for everyone. How can you tell if the candida diet is right for you? Ask yourself these questions, answer them honestly, and consider your answers carefully.

Do you often eat large amounts of starches, simple carbohydrates, and sugary foods? Do you feel intense cravings for these foods? After you eat them, do you feel bloated or sick, or gain weight even though you exercise—sometimes intensely? Do you find yourself trapped in your cycle of craving when it comes to these foods?

As you know already, the high-nutrient, low-carbohydrate, and healthy focus of the candida diet will assist you in breaking this cycle.

Do you have trouble keeping your blood sugar levels stable? Do you experience energy highs and then crashes throughout the day?

The candida diet will help you bring your system back in balance. By burning the right kinds of foods, you will avoid the blood sugar spikes and resulting insulin rise and fall that characterize blood sugar problems.

Are you experiencing fatigue, depression, a lack of energy, or a lack of motivation?

These are all common signs of candida buildup. Eliminating the foods that feed candida will actually provide you with more energy, even though it seems as if eating fewer carbohydrates might result in less energy. The end result will be more steady, slow-burning energy and far less fatigue.

Do you have autoimmune or inflammatory health problems?

People with autoimmune and/or inflammatory disorders are far more likely to suffer from candida buildup. Candida leaks into the bloodstream, causing the immune system to overreact; this exaggerated immune response is what drives candida sensitivity. While addressing the candida sensitivity may not cure your underlying autoimmune health issue, there is no question that it will stop candida buildup from exacerbating the problem. The candida diet also helps because it restricts foods that research shows increases intestinal permeability.

Do you have food allergies or sensitivities?

By eating whole, unprocessed foods, you eliminate additives, artificial flavorings, excitotoxins (chemicals that cause brain cells to become overexcited and fire uncontrollably), food coloring, sugars, preservatives, most added sodium, and most other unhealthy additions to your food. These all worsen food sensitivities.

Do you have digestive tract problems? Do you suffer from constipation, diarrhea, GERD, IBS, gas, bloating, or other digestive issues?

Candida sensitivity may be at the root of these issues. Eliminating foods that feed this fungus stops the problem where it starts.

If your answers to these questions signal to you that candida might be your problem, take this diet seriously. Give your body the chance it deserves to heal. If you are reading this book, you already know that you are in need of a serious, long-term solution.

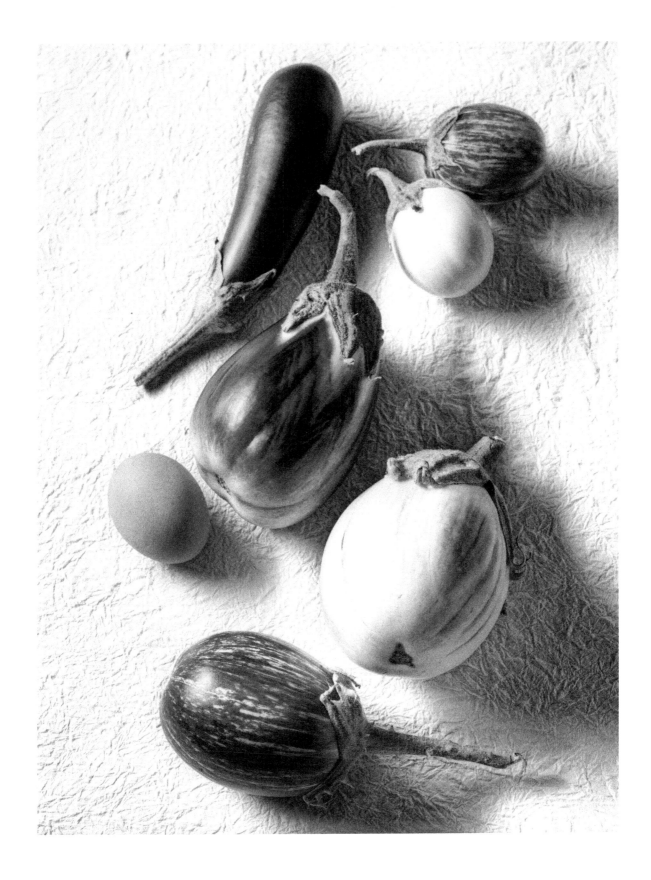

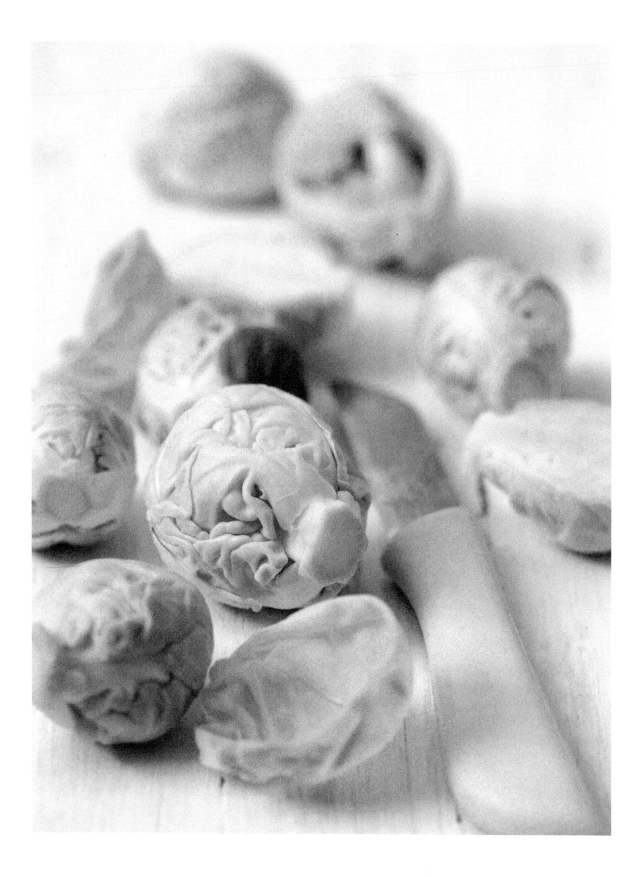

3

The Basics of the Candida Diet

Perhaps at this point you're concerned that eating to eliminate candida sensitivity is too challenging. Don't worry! This is something you can do. Yes, it requires some effort, but it will definitely get easier as you move forward. Take this opportunity to not only anticipate your own better health but also to get excited about the food you'll be preparing for yourself. With some creativity and thought, you can and will enjoy your new routine.

Foods to Enjoy

Beverages, Drinks, and Brews

- Chicory root coffee
- Freshly juiced vegetables on your safe list
- Tea brewed from anise, cinnamon, ginger, licorice, pau d'arco, or peppermint
- Water, plain or lightly flavored with lemon or cucumber

Brewed drinks are all antifungal and extremely beneficial to your digestive system. Chicory root is a natural prebiotic and can help your gut to rebalance itself with healthy flora. Cinnamon improves circulation, which also aids in digestion. Peppermint fights nausea. When juicing vegetables, choose leafy greens, which counteract cravings for sweets. They also contain enzymes that aid with digestion and improve kidney and liver function.

HOMEMADE BLENDER MAYONNAISE

Makes about 2 to 2¼ cups

2 EGG YOLKS, AT ROOM TEMPERATURE
1 WHOLE EGG, AT ROOM TEMPERATURE
1 TABLESPOON FRESHLY SQUEEZED LEMON JUICE, PLUS MORE IF NEEDED
1 TEASPOON DIJON MUSTARD
½ TEASPOON SEA SALT
PINCH FRESHLY GROUND WHITE PEPPER (OPTIONAL)
ABOUT 2 CUPS OLIVE OIL

1. Put the egg yolks, whole egg, lemon juice, mustard, salt, and white pepper (if using) in the blender. Blend at high speed for 10 seconds or more, until creamy.

2. Keep the blender running at a high speed and add the oil slowly, in a very thin stream. This is because mayonnaise is an emulsion, and you need to give the ingredients a chance to emulsify, or blend and thicken together, so that they won't fall apart and separate again. Add no more than 10 percent of the oil at first. Wait at least 30 seconds each time before adding any more oil to allow for emulsification.

3. When you see a notable thickening, add the rest of the oil in a thin stream, taking a break every few seconds and then continuing, and keeping the blender running. Each time you take a quick break, make sure all the oil is being absorbed by the mixture. You may not need the entire 2 cups, so be careful to stop when it the mixture looks like mayonnaise.

4. When you think it's finished, stop the blender and check it for taste and consistency. Adjust the salt, pepper, and lemon juice as needed. You may also add a small amount of lemon juice if your mayonnaise is too thick. If it is too thin, process it further, adding more oil as you did before.

5. Store the mayonnaise covered in the refrigerator for up to 1 week. Fresher eggs make mayonnaise that lasts longer.

Eggs

- Whole eggs
- Mayonnaise, homemade

Look for fresh eggs, and of course, organic if possible. Remember, if you cook them, cook using fats that are on your list. And don't miss the delicious, fresh taste of home-made mayonnaise!

If you need to maintain or gain weight while cleansing your body of candida overgrowth, you will have to take special care to take in enough calories to avoid weight loss. According to the Anti-Candida Diet Plan website, one of your best weapons against weight loss is healthy fat, such as that found in nuts, seeds, eggs, and avocados.

Fish

- Anchovies
- Herring
- Sardines
- Wild salmon

These varieties of fish (and unfortunately, no others) have levels of contaminants that are low enough for candida sufferers. Choose only fresh fish or fish canned and packed in water or olive oil.

Fruit

- Avocados
- Cranberries, unsweetened
- Lemons
- Limes
- Rhubarb, unsweetened

These fruits are safe during your cleansing period. After you rid your system of candida buildup and eliminate your symptoms, you may also reintroduce apples, blueberries, peaches, pears, pineapples, raspberries, and strawberries in small amounts.

Herbs and Spices

- Agrimony
- Andrographis
- Barberry
- Basil
- Bitter orange
- Black cumin
- Black pepper
- Black walnut
- Cinnamon
- Cloves
- Cumin
- Dill
- Echinacea
- Garlic
- Gentian
- Ginger
- Goldenseal
- Neem
- Oregano
- Oregon grape root
- Paprika
- Parsley
- Rosemary
- Thyme
- Wormwood

Many herbs and spices are natural antifungal agents, and some also act as anti-inflammatories. When you are on a limited diet, herbs and spices are your closest allies, adding flavor and dimension to your meals. Remember that one fresh tablespoon of herbs is equivalent to about one teaspoon of dried herbs.

Live Active Cultures

- Apple cider vinegar
- Kefir
- Kimchi
- Sauerkraut
- Yogurt with active cultures

The live cultures in these products help your body fight candida overgrowth and repopulate your gut with healthy bacteria. Live cultures in yogurt and other cultured foods will also restore the natural bacterial balance to your system.

Meats

- Beef
- Chicken
- Lamb
- Turkey

Eat only fresh meats. Avoid all processed, packed, smoked, vacuum-packed, and lunch meats. Choose organic meats whenever possible to minimize your intake of additives and preservatives.

Nuts and Seeds

- Almonds
- Coconut
- Flaxseed
- Hazelnuts
- Pecans
- Sunflower seeds
- Walnuts

These nuts and seeds are great for you and have a low enough mold content for you to safely enjoy them.

Oils and Fats

- Almond oil
- Butter
- Coconut oil
- Flaxseed oil
- Ghee
- Grapeseed oil
- Lard
- Macadamia oil
- Olive oil
- Red palm oil
- Sesame oil
- Sunflower oil
- Walnut oil

Coconut oil is a natural antifungal that you can drink as a supplement or cook with. Coconut oil contains three different fatty acids that fight candida without allowing the fungus to build up resistance: caprylic acid, capric acid, and lauric acid. Coconut oil also helps prevent candida buildup from recurring. You can add coconut oil to your diet by just eating one or two tablespoons each morning, eventually working up to five tablespoons a day. If you consume too much coconut oil, you will experience diarrhea and stomach cramps; if that happens, obviously reduce your dose. To receive maximum health benefits, buy organic, virgin coconut oil. As your body adjusts to a daily dose of coconut oil, get ready for not only a more successful battle against candida buildup but also shinier hair, healthier skin, lower cholesterol levels, and a tougher immune system.

These fats are all safe and healthy for you to use while fighting candida sensitivity and buildup. Regular (not extra-virgin) olive oil and coconut oil are best for everyday cooking, and coconut oil is better than olive oil at high heat. Extra-virgin olive oil smokes at high temperatures, so keep this in mind when planning your meals; it also has a stronger olive taste, if this matters to you. Many seed oils, including flaxseed oil, sunflower oil, and sesame oil, are not good for cooking but are lovely for making dressings and as condiments. Whenever you are able, use cold-pressed oils. This process preserves the nutrients of the nut, seed, or fruit from which the oil came.

Other Seasonings

- Apple cider vinegar
- Coconut aminos
- Garlic
- Lemon juice
- Olive leaf
- Onion
- Pesto, homemade
- Sea salt

Try making dressings by mixing olive oil or extra-virgin olive oil and apple cider vinegar or lemon juice; season your dressing simply with salt and pepper. If you aren't familiar with coconut aminos, it's basically coconut tree sap. You'll find it to be a fantastic alternative to soy sauce and a must for candida-free living. Look for it in health food stores and online.

HOMEMADE BASIL PESTO

Makes about 1 cup

1 CUP PACKED CHOPPED FRESH BASIL, STEMS REMOVED
¼ CUP OLIVE OIL
3 TEASPOONS FRESHLY SQUEEZED LEMON JUICE
4 TABLESPOONS PINE NUTS OR CHOPPED ALMONDS
4 GARLIC CLOVES
PINCH SEA SALT

1. Blend the basil, olive oil, lemon juice, pine nuts, garlic, and salt in a processor or blender until it is puréed.

2. If the pesto is too thick, add 1 to 2 tablespoons of warm water and blend again until smooth.

3. Store the pesto in a sealed container in the fridge for up to 2 weeks.

Sweeteners

- Stevia

This is your only totally safe choice. Remember, anything sweet gets its sweetness from something, and you must avoid sugars. Stevia is a safe source of sweetness—the only one—because it does not contain sugar in any form. But be careful: Some commercial stevia products mix in other ingredients, including other types of sweeteners; only 100 percent stevia is safe on a candida diet. That's why it's best to keep a supply of stevia on hand—not just at home but also at work, in your bag when you leave the house, in your gym bag, wherever you might be. This way you can treat yourself to the sweet taste you're missing by having some herbal tea wherever you are.

Vegetables

- Artichokes
- Asparagus
- Bok choy
- Broccoli

- Broccoli rabe
- Brussels sprouts
- Cabbage
- Carrots

- Cauliflower
- Celery
- Chard
- Cucumber
- Dandelion greens
- Eggplant
- Kale
- Leeks
- Lettuce
- Olives
- Onions
- Parsley
- Rutabagas
- Shallots
- Spinach
- Tomatoes
- Zucchini

Non-starchy vegetables are perfect as you eliminate the candida buildup from your body. These vegetables help you curb cravings for sweets and starve the candida. Eat these vegetables grilled, steamed, or, for the most nutritional impact, raw. For all these vegetables, choose fresh produce, and organic whenever you can to minimize your exposure to pesticides and other contaminants. Olives are an acceptable treat as long as they are not cured using vinegar.

Whole Grains

- Buckwheat
- Millet
- Oat bran
- Quinoa

These grains are high in fiber, which helps your digestive tract get rid of candida waste products and otherwise keep everything moving. Also remember to use flours made from only these whole grains.

Special Healthy Practices to Keep in Mind

Use antimicrobial and antifungal herbs and foods to your best advantage. Agrimony, *Andrographis,* barberry, bitter orange, black cumin, black walnut, cloves, dandelion, echinacea, garlic, gentian, golden seal, neem, olive leaf, onions, Oregon grape, pau d'arco, rhubarb, thyme, and wormwood are all antiparasitic, anti-infective, and protect the liver. Include them in your diet fresh or in high-quality supplements that contain no additives.

Restore the healthy balance of normal bacterial flora in your body with probiotics. Take *Lactobacillus acidophilus* and *Bifidobacteria bifidus* supplements every day. When you do, you will notice a reduction in symptoms such as bloating, constipation, thrush, and even more traditional candidiasis symptoms.

Fight leaky gut and repair the integrity of your gastrointestinal membranes with foods rich in glutamine. Eat glutamine-rich foods such as Brussels sprouts, celery, dandelion greens, lettuce, parsley, and spinach to counteract leaky gut symptoms and work toward strengthening your GI system permanently.

Use healthy equipment too. Make sure your nonstick cooking spray is made with one of your safe oils, and contains no artificial propellants or other additives.

Foods to Avoid

Additives and Preservatives

- Anything you can't identify or pronounce
- Citric acid

Although the natural form of citric acid that is found in lemons and limes is fine, the manufactured, additive form of citric acid is yeast-based. Other food additives and preservatives can and frequently do disrupt healthy intestinal flora and cause an imbalance in the GI system.

Alcohol

- Beer
- Hard cider
- Liquor and spirits
- Wine

Alcohol is high in sugars and, therefore, instant food for candida. It's also tough on your body and your immune system. When alcohol enters your system, it is immediately metabolized, with up to 20 percent of it entering your bloodstream directly from the stomach. In other words, alcohol acts like instant sugar. To make matters worse, alcohol is either fermented, sugar-based, or both. Avoid it no matter what.

Artificial Sweeteners

Even non-caloric sweeteners like aspartame can cause blood sugar to spike in ways similar to sugar, and may also be a carcinogen. Although some research seems to indicate that xylitol is safe for candida sufferers, because the facts are not 100 percent clear on this point, we recommend stevia as the one absolutely established safe sweetener for candida sufferers.

GMO stands for "genetically modified organism"—foods that have been changed in some way by genetic engineering techniques. The goal of creating GMOs has traditionally been to improve the ability of crops to resist drought or pest attacks and increase crop yields. Critics say these altered foods have been introduced without sufficient research into their safety. They are banned in some countries, although they are approved in many others, including the United States. The bottom line is that we still do not know for sure if foods made from GMO crops are safe. For a diet that emphasizes natural foods, such as this one, it is best to avoid GMOs.

Beans and Legumes

- Beans
- Chickpeas
- Peanuts
- Soy products, including tofu

These foods are difficult to digest and relatively higher in carbohydrates than other foods, so they cannot be eaten during the initial cleanse portion of the diet, despite the fact that they are generally healthy foods. You may return legumes to your diet later in small portions. Unfortunately, all soy products are off the list, as the majority of soy products are GMO.

Caffeine Beverages

- Black tea
- Coffee
- Diet soda
- Energy drinks
- Green tea
- Soda

Caffeine causes your blood sugar to spike and burdens your immune system. Even beverages that have been decaffeinated contain some caffeine. Coffee and some kinds of tea also contain mold, which should be completely avoided.

Condiments

- Ketchup
- Horseradish
- Mayonnaise, commercially prepared
- Mustard, commercially prepared
- Relish

- Salad dressings, commercially prepared
- Soy sauce
- Tomato paste
- Tomato sauce, commercially prepared

All of these commercially prepared sauces and dressings contain high amounts of hidden sugars. For an alternative salad dressing, try a simple olive oil and lemon juice dressing. Dry mustard from your spice rack is also fine, as is homemade mayonnaise (page 30).

Dairy Products

- Buttermilk
- Cheese
- Cottage cheese
- Cream
- Ice cream
- Milk
- Sour cream

Almost all dairy should be avoided (the exceptions are listed in Foods to Enjoy). Milk and anything else containing lactose must be avoided because lactose is a kind of sugar. Kefir and yogurt are better choices; almost all of the lactose disappears as they ferment.

Fats and Oils

- Canola oil
- Corn oil
- Peanut oil
- Soybean oil

Canola oil, corn oil, and peanut oil are all contaminated with mold. Most soybeans used in soy oil are GMO. Refer to the safe fats and oils listed in Foods to Enjoy for exceptions.

Fish and Seafood

All seafood and most fish are far too high in immune system–compromising heavy metals and toxins to be safe (the exceptions are listed in Foods to Enjoy). Salmon *must* be wild-caught because farmed varieties usually contain high levels of PCBs, mercury, and other carcinogens.

Fruit

- Canned
- Dried
- Fresh
- Juiced

Fruit is too high in natural sugars to be eaten while eliminating candida buildup. Some fresh fruit in limited amounts may be introduced later. Dried fruit, fruit juice, and canned fruit, in particular, have very high sugar content and must be avoided. Some melons, such as cantaloupe, also have moldy rinds, and discarding the rind does not mean avoiding the mold altogether. An occasional spritz of lemon juice as a flavoring is fine, though. Just be sure to use the real thing, not a bottled juice.

Grains and Gluten

- Barley
- Corn
- Oats
- Rice
- Rye
- Spelt
- Wheat

Candida overgrowth and gluten sensitivity go hand in hand, and many grains—especially popcorn—are contaminated with mold. Avoid all the grains listed here, and any product made with flour from these grains. Obviously, too, any yeast bread is off limits because of the yeast contained in it.

Meats

- Canned, cured, processed, smoked, or vacuum-packed meat
- Lunch or deli meats
- Pork and any pork products

Processed meats contain additives such as dextrose nitrates and sulfates, not to mention sugars. Pork is dangerous for those with digestive problems because it contains retroviruses that survive cooking.

Mushrooms and Fungi

Most mushrooms and fungi are harmful if you suffer from candida buildup and sensitivity, although shiitake, maitake, and reishi mushrooms are exceptions. These mushrooms actually boost the immune system and help protect against infection, including candida.

Nuts

- Cashews
- Peanuts
- Pistachios

These kinds of nuts are very moldy. Stick to the nuts on the "safe" list. This means anything made with these nut butters or containing even small amounts of any of these nuts should be avoided.

Sweeteners

- Agave
- Brown sugar
- Granulated sugar
- Honey
- Maple syrup
- Molasses
- Rice syrup

Remember that processed foods are filled with hidden sugars. Be careful. Always read labels. But even whole foods can contain added honey or maple syrup as a flavoring. Assume restaurant food has far more sweeteners than you think.

Vegetables

- Beets
- Carrots
- Parsnips
- Peas
- Potatoes
- Sweet potatoes
- Yams

These are very healthy foods, but they are also high in carbohydrates. They may be reintroduced one at a time only when your cleanse is over and your candida overgrowth is under control.

Vinegar

Because vinegars are made using yeast cultures and can cause inflammation in your gut, they must be avoided. This is true of all vinegars except unfiltered apple cider vinegar.

Shopping While on the Candida Diet

Once you commit to avoiding candida-fueling foods in your diet, you must relearn how to shop for food. This is primarily because so much of the food in the supermarket is unsafe for candida sufferers. All sorts of prepared foods—even "health" foods—are off the list, so it's important to have a nice store of fresh, "safe" foods at home. Sticking to your new diet is so much easier that way, even when you don't have time to shop or look for new recipes or new ways to eat familiar foods.

Here are some easy tips to help you maintain your kitchen as an anti-candida zone.

Shop Frequently for Small Amounts of Fresh Food

It always feels productive to get ahead on a task, but don't do this when it comes to your candida shopping list. Resist the urge to stock up. If you need basics that last on a shelf,

WHAT ARE THE HEALTH BENEFITS OF APPLE CIDER VINEGAR?

- **Blood pressure and heart health:** People who ate oil and apple cider vinegar dressing on salads five to six times a week had lower rates of heart disease than people who didn't, according to WebMD. However, it's not clear that the apple cider vinegar was the reason.

- **Blood sugar levels:** Apple cider vinegar may help lower blood glucose levels. A 2007 study published in *Diabetes Care* of eleven people with type 2 diabetes found that taking two tablespoons of apple cider vinegar before bed lowered glucose levels in the morning by 4 to 6 percent.

- **Cancer:** WebMD reports that some laboratory studies have found that apple cider vinegar may be able to kill or slow the growth of cancer cells.

- **Cholesterol:** The *British Journal of Nutrition* published a 2006 study showing that apple cider vinegar may help lower cholesterol.

- **Weight loss:** Apple cider vinegar is often used as an aid in weight loss and may help people feel full.

you may absolutely stock up. However, even fairly long-lasting items such as grains and jarred foods should be as fresh as you can get them. Particularly when you're trying to beat candida, you need to choose the freshest options available, whenever possible. Fresh foods degrade over time, losing some of their nutrient value—and much of their taste.

Once you're in the habit of making small, frequent trips to the market, you will also find that you are far more likely to shop according to your cleanse rules. Visiting the meat, fish, and produce counters at your local market daily or every other day will enable you to choose what looks best and appeals to you right now. It also helps you avoid waste.

Patronize Stores That Reliably Offer Organic Foods

This habit gives you easier access to organic choices, of course. It also enables you to locate more unusual and alternative food choices that candida sufferers sometimes have trouble finding, such as kefir, flaxseed, more unusual grains and products made from them (millet crackers, for example), and more exotic oils and products made from them (coconut oil cooking spray, for example).

Become a Habitual Label Reader

There is probably no other single tip that is more important for your candida cleanse. *Never* assume you know what's in something, just because you know what the dish itself is. It doesn't matter how many times you have eaten that food, or how sure you are that this particular dish is wonderful for your health. Committing yourself to eliminating your candida buildup and living successfully with candida sensitivity means being sure you are preventing all sources of candida from reentering your body. You cannot leave this to chance.

If there is anything on the label that you're unsure of, do not buy it. If there are any ingredients in a food item that you can't pronounce, put it down. If something you want to eat contains even a very small amount of a food, additive, or ingredient that you cannot consume, do not eat it. If you follow these rules closely, you will find yourself rejecting almost every processed food item—and that's exactly what you should be doing.

Eating Out While on the Candida Diet

With any cleanse or new food regime, eating out is challenging initially. It's not impossible, though, and after a short period of time it will get a lot easier. Keep in mind these central habits and you will be able to dine out successfully whenever you want or need to.

See Dining Out as Business as Usual, Not a Splurge

It's easy to see eating out as a special occasion—and sometimes it is. Even so, don't get into that mindset as a matter of habit when you choose what you'll eat. That outlook makes it easier to stray from the safe foods list. Instead, learn to see eating out as another way of eating—whether you are at home, a guest in someone else's house, or otherwise being a traveler searching for safe foods. Keep a "safety first" mindset as you look over menus and consider your choices.

Ask Questions—Lots of Them

Any food server worth their salt takes no issue with you asking questions about the menu; it's their job to know the answers—or to get them. In fact, it absolves them of guilt in many situations, especially now that so many people are known to have special needs stemming from allergies, food sensitivities, diabetes, and other problems. Speak up before you order! Here are some examples.

If you have a taste for grilled salmon, make sure it's wild-caught. You must also find out what they prepare the fish with before it's grilled. There is virtually no chance the salmon doesn't have some kind of preparation or marinade on it, and most of these feed candida. However, there is also just about a 100 percent certainty that the chef has olive oil, salt, and pepper. If whoever is cooking your salmon simply brushes it in olive oil, sprinkles it with salt and pepper, and grills it, you will be perfectly safe eating it with a lemon wedge on the side.

Bring Your Own Extras If You Need To

You should bring things like stevia with you. If you are sure you're going to need coconut aminos at a Chinese restaurant, bring them. If there are other foods that you find key to your success, bring them!

Take Advantage of Accommodations for Allergies and Similar Situations

Everyone, especially anyone working in or running a restaurant, is much more aware of food allergies today than they were twenty years ago. Treat your cleanse diet as if you are dealing with multiple food allergies. This isn't far from the mark, after all; you are avoiding foods that have made you seriously ill over time. Talk to your server and, if needed, the chef, about your food sensitivities and take advantage of their skill and creativity. You may be pleasantly surprised at the choices they come up with for you. Remember, these are people who are genuinely invested in your enjoyment of the meal and they will do what they can to ensure it.

When You Have a Choice, Pick a Healthy Restaurant

When your sister calls and asks if you'd rather go to the Bread Bistro or the Healthy Green Cafe, make the choice that makes the most sense for your cleanse (definitely not the Bread Bistro!). If you're not sure which option is best, take five minutes and research it online. This will save you so much trouble and frustration later. If you eat out for business or pleasure frequently, you can even maintain a "safe" list of good restaurants for when it's your turn to host or choose.

Moving to Maintenance Mode

Remember, you will probably always require a much healthier, low-sugar diet than you lived on before. Candida buildup is a problem that can keep coming back, and candida sensitivity is something that stays with you for life. In the long term you will need to avoid:

- Eating junk food in significant amounts again
- Eating large amounts of sugar—even as it naturally occurs in fruit
- Antibiotics, unless they are medically necessary

You will need to follow these rules consistently, and for a long time—possibly for life. Candida is a fast-growing, opportunistic fungus that will take advantage of any opportunity for growth that you give it.

Once you are no longer experiencing most candida buildup symptoms, you may begin to reintroduce certain foods, but only one at a time. This way, you can isolate any food that causes you problems and eliminate it from your diet, if necessary. It may take as many as eight to twelve weeks for you to feel well enough to graduate to maintenance mode, and it may take longer, based on your starting point and overall health.

Beans and Legumes

- All legumes except peanuts, soybeans, and soy products

These foods are difficult to digest and relatively higher in carbohydrates than other foods, so they cannot be eaten during the initial cleanse phase of the diet, despite the fact that they are healthy foods. You may return legumes to your diet later in small portions. You may not consume soybeans or soy products at any time on this diet, because of the concern about GMO crops. Peanuts tend to attract mold, and so are also off the list.

Fruit

- Apples
- Blueberries
- Peaches
- Pears
- Pineapples
- Raspberries
- Strawberries

Reintroduce these in small amounts.

Vegetables

- Beets
- Carrots
- Parsnips
- Peas
- Potatoes
- Sweet potatoes
- Yams

These are very healthy foods, but they are high in carbohydrates. They may be reintroduced one at a time only once your cleanse is over and your candida overgrowth is under control.

Ten Tips for Cleansing Success

1. **Don't forget to exercise.** The candida diet is not a regular diet designed to help you lose weight, so people often forget the exercise component. Exercise is the foundation for general good health and can be crucial when combating candida symptoms. Exercise moderately at least four times per week by walking, biking, weight training, dancing, or playing a favorite sport. Some of the candida-related benefits attributed to exercising include:
   - A stimulated lymphatic system, which encourages waste, fungi, and bacteria to be removed from your systems
   - An unclogged liver so that your body can effectively detox and flush candida out
   - A clearer mind and lessening of candida-related fatigue
   - A general feeling of wellness, which can combat depression

   Consult your doctor before embarking on any exercise program, especially if you are overweight or have other health concerns.

2. **Take small steps.** The candida diet is a very big adjustment for many people because it prohibits and restricts many of the foods that make up a huge portion of the average diet. Eliminating frequently consumed foods cold turkey can be physically overwhelming and mentally unsustainable, so it is a better strategy to follow a step-by-step elimination process to ensure success. Remove major detox foods first, such as sugar, so that withdrawal problems don't become too uncomfortable. Depending on your consumption level of these foods, you might find yourself suffering from headaches and nausea. These unpleasant withdrawal symptoms can sideline your diet if combined with quitting coffee, processed foods, gluten, and other foods. So take one group at a time, and when you are comfortable with the exclusion, try another group. The candida diet is a lifetime commitment; spending some time easing into it will not cause further damage.

3. **Be patient with yourself.** As with any important change in life, it can be difficult to be patient during the process. Once you make a decision to embrace a new diet, you want to follow it perfectly right away, with no roadblocks or regression to old habits. Accept the fact you might fall off the diet wagon at some point in the journey. Relapsing is fine, and all you need to do is dust off and start your diet again. These small lapses should never create self-defeating thoughts or be used as an excuse to binge. Depending on how long you have been following the candida diet, you might find these lapses create a resurgence of symptoms. These physical reminders should be motivation to get back on the plan and stay on it for your health.

4. **Adjust your thinking to include the changes you need to make.** One of the problem with following the candida diet is that it restricts many foods that are mainstream choices for almost everyone else around you. Sugar, wheat products, alcohol, caffeine, and a plethora of other foods are found in every pantry, fridge, and on most plates. Instead of feeling a bit like an outcast and that you are being punished, it is much more accurate to perceive yourself as someone who has learned the secret to good health. For example, refined sugar is not good for you, or for anyone. Simple sugar is addictive, destructive, and can lead to diabetes, obesity, and other diseases and health hazards. Change your thinking about denying yourself this poison and other unhealthy foods and embrace the positive changes in your body now that you're eating healthier.

5. **Find a like-minded community.** There is a very good chance that your family, friends, and coworkers will not be overly supportive of the drastic lifestyle choices you will make following this diet. Most people are simply not aware of the destructive power food can have on their health and will see your changes as either inconvenient or simply over the top. This negative feedback can be crippling and cause you to question your commitment. Find support from a therapist or community of people who are following the same plan as you in the quest to live better. You can find these people online, in health food stores, at local farmers' markets, and by searching community calendars.

6. **Purge your house of temptations.** This could be difficult if you have other household members who are eating a regular diet. Be realistic about your environment purge. You might want to place your family on the same diet as you or at least a modified version so that they also enjoy the benefits of a healthier lifestyle. At a minimum, remove any processed foods and all the products in the house that contain refined sugar. This will help limit your temptations, and your family can still enjoy bread, dried fruit, and dairy. Make sure those choices are healthy versions, as well, to support your family's health.

7. **Always be prepared when out of the house.** There will be a point in your cleanse when you eat out again, go to a family event, or just go to work. The candida diet is for life in most cases, so it is unrealistic and emotionally unhealthy to assume you will never be tempted again. The most important part of going out is to have a plan. For example, most restaurants have their menus posted online, so pick your meal in advance and know what modifications need to be made to your dish. When going to a family event, simply call up the person who is hosting it and explain your diet. If they cannot accommodate your needs, pack up your own meal and bring it with you. Packing a lunch from home is also a great strategy for eating at work. There are always healthy choices in any situation if you are willing to look for them.

8. **Choose organic produce for your diet.** Eating organic produce seems like a healthy choice for anyone, but it can be particularly important for someone suffering from candida issues. Organic produce does not have the same chemicals, pesticides, toxins, and additives that are found in commercially grown food. These contaminants can wreak havoc on your system, so it is better to avoid them whenever possible. If you live in an area that does not offer a wide range of organic options or your budget does not support this choice, wash your produce thoroughly in a water and vinegar solution to remove the majority of the surface contaminants.

9. **Look at the rest of your life for harmful products.** When purging your fridge and pantry of all the foods that are not recommended on the plan, also take a hard look at other aspects of your life. Environmental toxins can also negatively impact your health. Remove products containing chemicals and harmful additives, such as shampoos, makeup, and cleaning supplies, including laundry soaps and air fresheners. Choose organic products that have natural ingredients, because what you expose your "outside" to can be as important as what you put inside your body.

10. **Have a weekly treat to combat feelings of deprivation.** This is not a license to consume a whole cake, but rather permission to enjoy an indulgence that is not too far off the list of allowed foods. If you are completely cut off from treats, it can become an obsession and lead to a real leap into destructive behavior. Savor a bowl of rice-based ice cream, a banana, or a mango. Pay attention to your body's reaction and adjust your choice if they cause symptoms. Life is for living and enjoying special moments, so find a treat that works and fall into the experience of eating it with blissful intent.

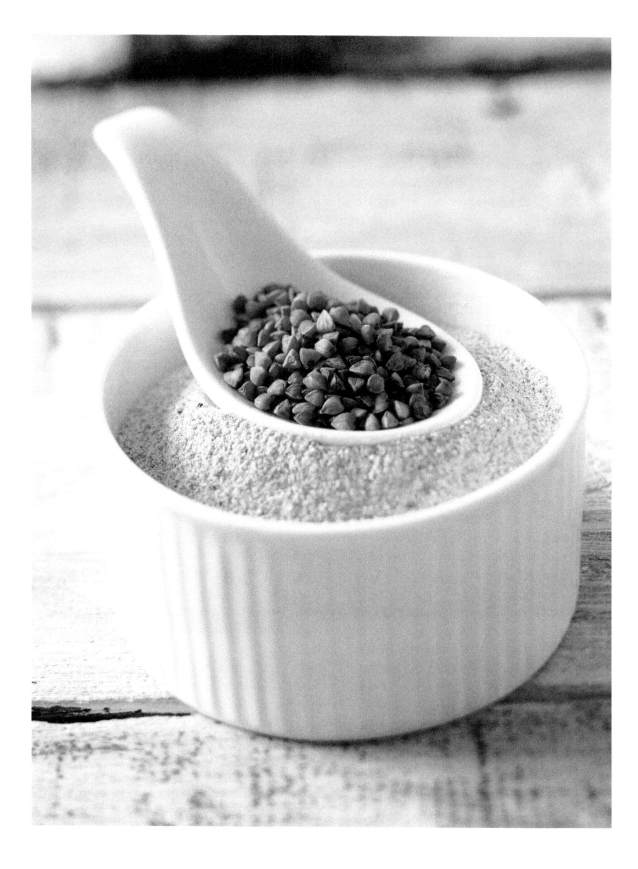

4

Cleansing Meal Plans

Let's take a closer look at how the candida diet will work from day to day. This chapter has both a thirty-day and a ninety-day cleanse diet. From Day 1 through Day 30 (or 90), each day will include a breakfast, midmorning snack, lunch, midday snack, dinner, and dessert. In other words, you can keep yourself both healthy and satisfied. Both these longer plans are centered on the cleanse stage, which may vary in length for each person.

Finally, you will find a seven-day meal plan for your maintenance mode. This will help you in transitioning to the maintenance stage of your candida diet, after your candida buildup symptoms have abated.

You will find recipes for all the dishes in these meal plans in part 2 of this book.

Keep in mind that these meal plans are simply tools for understanding and personalizing your candida diet. You don't need to follow them exactly from day to day. Mix and match whatever meals you want to. These meal plans are a starting point for you to participate in the creation of your own personalized plan to eliminate candida buildup from your body without being concerned about your health or nutrition lacking in some way.

Thirty-Day Cleanse Meal Plan

The transition to maintenance mode on this meal plan begins on Day 25. But if you feel you are ready to make the transition before that, by all means skip ahead to Day 25 and start adding in some new healthy foods. If, after twenty-five days, you still don't feel able to make the transition, pick up the ninety-day meal plan. Listen to your body and don't rush yourself.

Day 1

BREAKFAST Coconut-Almond Waffles
SNACK Quinoa-Sesame Buckwheat Crackers
LUNCH Almond Butter Bread
SNACK Oven-Roasted Onion-Garlic Dip
DINNER Vegetable "Fried Rice"
DESSERT Fresh Mint Bars

Day 2

BREAKFAST Steak and Sunny-Side Up Eggs with Skillet Tomatoes
SNACK Cayenne-Spiced Walnuts
LUNCH Kale Salad with Toasted Walnuts and Eggs
SNACK Trail Mix
DINNER Lime-Garlic Chicken with Avocado Salsa
DESSERT Chai-Coconut Ice Pops

Day 3

BREAKFAST Zucchini-Herb Frittata
SNACK Oven-Roasted Onion-Garlic Dip
LUNCH Avocado-Basil Chicken Salad
SNACK Roasted Radicchio with Thyme
DINNER Kid-Friendly Chicken Fingers
DESSERT I Scream for Vanilla Ice Cream

Day 4

BREAKFAST Poached Eggs with Quinoa and Spinach
SNACK Spicy Baked Chicken Wings
LUNCH Spinach-Celeriac Soup
SNACK Chili-Lime Jicama with Diced Cucumbers
DINNER Grilled Beef Skewers with Zucchini
DESSERT Chocolate "Milkshake"

Day 5

BREAKFAST Baked Eggs with Kale and Yogurt
SNACK Puffed Quinoa Treats
LUNCH Grilled Chicken and Arugula Salad
SNACK Quinoa with Fresh Herb Vinaigrette
DINNER Salmon with Garlic and Ginger
DESSERT Nutty Coconut Bark

Day 6

BREAKFAST Steak and Sunny-Side Up
Eggs with Skillet Tomatoes
SNACK Chili-Lime Jicama with Diced
Cucumbers
LUNCH Classic Egg Drop Soup
SNACK Garlicky Mixed Bitter Greens
DINNER Grilled Sirloin with
Garlic Butter
DESSERT Fresh Mint Bars

Day 7

BREAKFAST Coconut-Almond Waffles
SNACK Trail Mix
LUNCH Grilled Skirt Steak Arugula
Salad with Cilantro-Lime Vinaigrette
SNACK Oven-Roasted Onion-Garlic Dip
DINNER Garlic and Rosemary
Chicken Thighs
DESSERT Chai-Coconut Ice Pops

Day 8

BREAKFAST Poached Eggs with Quinoa
and Spinach
SNACK Gingery Brussels Sprouts
LUNCH Poached Salmon and
Avocado Salad
SNACK Spicy Baked Chicken Wings
DINNER Lentil Curry with Spinach
DESSERT I Scream for Vanilla
Ice Cream

Day 9

BREAKFAST Zucchini-Herb Frittata
SNACK Garlicky Mixed Bitter Greens
LUNCH Cream of Roasted
Cauliflower Soup
SNACK Puffed Quinoa Treats
DINNER Coconut Chicken with
Bok Choy
DESSERT Chocolate "Milkshake"

Day 10

BREAKFAST Poached Eggs with Quinoa
and Spinach
SNACK Roasted Radicchio with Thyme
LUNCH Tomato Florentine Soup
SNACK Gingery Brussels Sprouts
DINNER Spicy Chicken Patties
DESSERT Nutty Coconut Bark

Day 11

BREAKFAST Baked Eggs with Kale
and Yogurt
SNACK Quinoa with Fresh Herb
Vinaigrette
LUNCH Kale Salad with Toasted
Walnuts and Eggs
SNACK Quinoa-Sesame Buckwheat
Crackers
DINNER Herb-Roasted Turkey
Tenderloin
DESSERT Fresh Mint Bars

Day 12

BREAKFAST Steak and Sunny-Side Up Eggs with Skillet Tomatoes
SNACK Quinoa-Sesame Buckwheat Crackers
LUNCH Avocado-Basil Chicken Salad
SNACK Cayenne-Spiced Walnuts
DINNER Lemony Pot Roast
DESSERT Chai-Coconut Ice Pops

Day 13

BREAKFAST Coconut-Almond Waffles
SNACK Cayenne-Spiced Walnuts
LUNCH Almond Butter Bread
SNACK Trail Mix
DINNER Poached Salmon with Warm Tomatoes
DESSERT I Scream for Vanilla Ice Cream

Day 14

BREAKFAST Poached Eggs with Quinoa and Spinach
SNACK Oven-Roasted Onion-Garlic Dip
LUNCH Poached Salmon and Avocado Salad
SNACK Roasted Radicchio with Thyme
DINNER Poached Salmon with Warm Tomatoes
DESSERT Chocolate "Milkshake"

Day 15

BREAKFAST Zucchini-Herb Frittata
SNACK Spicy Baked Chicken Wings
LUNCH Grilled Skirt Steak Arugula Salad with Cilantro-Lime Vinaigrette
SNACK Chili-Lime Jicama with Diced Cucumbers
DINNER Grilled Moroccan Salmon
DESSERT Nutty Coconut Bark

Day 16

BREAKFAST Poached Eggs with Quinoa and Spinach
SNACK Puffed Quinoa Treats
LUNCH Grilled Chicken and Arugula Salad
SNACK Quinoa with Fresh Herb Vinaigrette
DINNER Pan-Seared Herring with Lime and Pepper
DESSERT Fresh Mint Bars

Day 17

BREAKFAST Baked Eggs with Kale and Yogurt
SNACK Chili-Lime Jicama with Diced Cucumbers
LUNCH Classic Egg Drop Soup
SNACK Garlicky Mixed Bitter Greens
DINNER Slow-Roasted Lamb Shoulder with Lemons
DESSERT Chai-Coconut Ice Pops

Day 18

BREAKFAST Steak and Sunny-Side Up
Eggs with Skillet Tomatoes
SNACK Spicy Baked Chicken Wings
LUNCH Spinach-Celeriac Soup
SNACK Trail Mix
DINNER Lamb Vindaloo
DESSERT I Scream for Vanilla
Ice Cream

Day 19

BREAKFAST Coconut-Almond Waffles
SNACK Gingery Brussels Sprouts
LUNCH Avocado-Basil Chicken Salad
SNACK Roasted Radicchio with Thyme
DINNER Vegetable "Fried Rice"
DESSERT Chocolate "Milkshake"

Day 20

BREAKFAST Poached Eggs with Quinoa
and Spinach
SNACK Garlicky Mixed Bitter Greens
LUNCH Almond Butter Bread
SNACK Cayenne-Spiced Walnuts
DINNER Lime-Garlic Chicken with
Avocado Salsa
DESSERT Nutty Coconut Bark

Day 21

BREAKFAST Zucchini-Herb Frittata
SNACK Gingery Brussels Sprouts
LUNCH Cream of Roasted
Cauliflower Soup
SNACK Puffed Quinoa Treats
DINNER Kid-Friendly Chicken Fingers
DESSERT Fresh Mint Bars

Day 22

BREAKFAST Poached Eggs with Quinoa
and Spinach
SNACK Chili-Lime Jicama with Diced
Cucumbers
LUNCH Kale Salad with Toasted
Walnuts and Eggs
SNACK Quinoa-Sesame Buckwheat
Crackers
DINNER Grilled Beef Skewers
with Zucchini
DESSERT Chai-Coconut Ice Pops

Day 23

BREAKFAST Baked Eggs with Kale
and Yogurt
SNACK Quinoa-Sesame Buckwheat
Crackers
LUNCH Grilled Skirt Steak Arugula
Salad with Cilantro-Lime Vinaigrette
SNACK Spicy Baked Chicken Wings
DINNER Salmon with Garlic and Ginger
DESSERT I Scream for Vanilla
Ice Cream

Day 24

BREAKFAST Steak and Sunny-Side Up Eggs with Skillet Tomatoes
SNACK Cayenne-Spiced Walnuts
LUNCH Grilled Chicken and Arugula Salad
SNACK Trail Mix
DINNER Garlic and Rosemary Chicken Thighs
DESSERT Chocolate "Milkshake"

Day 25

Transition to
Maintenance Mode Begins

BREAKFAST Coconut-Almond Waffles
SNACK Berry Skewers with Chia-Yogurt Dip
LUNCH Beef and Vegetable Stew
SNACK Quinoa-Sesame Buckwheat Crackers
DINNER Salmon with Garlic and Ginger
DESSERT Warm Apple Bake with Streusel Topping

Day 26

BREAKFAST Blueberry-Lemon Pancakes
SNACK Carrots with Gremolata
LUNCH Quinoa Salad with Roasted Sweet Potato and Apples
SNACK Roasted Radicchio with Thyme
DINNER Turkey Cabbage Rolls
DESSERT Strawberry Shortcake

Day 27

BREAKFAST Quinoa Porridge with Cardamom, Almonds, and Sliced Pear
SNACK Roasted Ginger-Cumin Chickpeas
LUNCH Kale Salad with Toasted Walnuts and Eggs
SNACK Puffed Quinoa Treats
DINNER Roasted Chicken with Pears
DESSERT Almond-Chocolate Truffles

Day 28

BREAKFAST Zucchini-Herb Frittata
SNACK Berry Savory Ants on a Log
LUNCH Mexican-Spiced Tomato and White Bean Soup
SNACK Mashed Parsnips and Apples
DINNER Herbed Chicken with White Beans
DESSERT Mixed-Berry Slushie

Day 29

BREAKFAST Sweetie Pie Smoothie
SNACK Roasted Beet and Garlic
"Hummus"
LUNCH Chicken and Sweet Potato Soup
with Collard Greens
SNACK Spicy Baked Chicken Wings
DINNER Grilled Beef Skewers with
Zucchini
DESSERT I Scream for Vanilla
Ice Cream

Day 30

BREAKFAST Coconut Millet with Cacao
and Raspberries
SNACK Roasted Eggplant Tapenade
LUNCH Grilled Chicken and
Arugula Salad
SNACK Coconut-Lime Sweet Potatoes
DINNER Lemony Pot Roast
DESSERT Chocolate "Milkshake"

Ninety-Day Cleanse Meal Plan

The transition to maintenance mode on this meal plan begins on Day 77. But if you feel you are ready to make the transition before that, by all means skip ahead to Day 77 and start adding in some new healthy foods.

Day 1

BREAKFAST Coconut-Almond Waffles
SNACK Quinoa-Sesame Buckwheat Crackers
LUNCH Almond Butter Bread
SNACK Oven-Roasted Onion-Garlic Dip
DINNER Vegetable "Fried Rice"
DESSERT Fresh Mint Bars

Day 2

BREAKFAST Poached Eggs with Quinoa and Spinach
SNACK Cayenne-Spiced Walnuts
LUNCH Kale Salad with Toasted Walnuts and Eggs
SNACK Trail Mix
DINNER Lime-Garlic Chicken with Avocado Salsa
DESSERT Chai-Coconut Ice Pops

Day 3

BREAKFAST Zucchini-Herb Frittata
SNACK Oven-Roasted Onion-Garlic Dip
LUNCH Avocado-Basil Chicken Salad
SNACK Roasted Radicchio with Thyme
DINNER Kid-Friendly Chicken Fingers
DESSERT I Scream for Vanilla Ice Cream

Day 4

BREAKFAST Poached Eggs with Quinoa and Spinach
SNACK Spicy Baked Chicken Wings
LUNCH Spinach-Celeriac Soup
SNACK Chili-Lime Jicama with Diced Cucumbers
DINNER Grilled Beef Skewers with Zucchini
DESSERT Chocolate "Milkshake"

Day 5

BREAKFAST Baked Eggs with Kale and Yogurt
SNACK Puffed Quinoa Treats
LUNCH Grilled Chicken and Arugula Salad
SNACK Quinoa with Fresh Herb Vinaigrette
DINNER Salmon with Garlic and Ginger
DESSERT Nutty Coconut Bark

Day 6

BREAKFAST Steak and Sunny-Side Up Eggs with Skillet Tomatoes
SNACK Chili-Lime Jicama with Diced Cucumbers
LUNCH Classic Egg Drop Soup
SNACK Garlicky Mixed Bitter Greens
DINNER Grilled Sirloin with Garlic Butter
DESSERT Fresh Mint Bars

Day 7

BREAKFAST Coconut-Almond Waffles
SNACK Trail Mix
LUNCH Grilled Skirt Steak Arugula Salad with Cilantro-Lime Vinaigrette
SNACK Oven-Roasted Onion-Garlic Dip
DINNER Garlic and Rosemary Chicken Thighs
DESSERT Chai-Coconut Ice Pops

Day 8

BREAKFAST Poached Eggs with Quinoa and Spinach
SNACK Gingery Brussels Sprouts
LUNCH Poached Salmon and Avocado Salad
SNACK Spicy Baked Chicken Wings
DINNER Lentil Curry with Spinach
DESSERT I Scream for Vanilla Ice Cream

Day 9

BREAKFAST Zucchini-Herb Frittata
SNACK Garlicky Mixed Bitter Greens
LUNCH Cream of Roasted Cauliflower Soup
SNACK Puffed Quinoa Treats
DINNER Coconut Chicken with Bok Choy
DESSERT Chocolate "Milkshake"

Day 10

BREAKFAST Poached Eggs with Quinoa and Spinach
SNACK Roasted Radicchio with Thyme
LUNCH Tomato Florentine Soup
SNACK Gingery Brussels Sprouts
DINNER Spicy Chicken Patties
DESSERT Nutty Coconut Bark

Day 11

BREAKFAST Baked Eggs with Kale and Yogurt
SNACK Quinoa with Fresh Herb Vinaigrette
LUNCH Kale Salad with Toasted Walnuts and Eggs
SNACK Quinoa-Sesame Buckwheat Crackers
DINNER Herb-Roasted Turkey Tenderloin
DESSERT Fresh Mint Bars

Day 12

BREAKFAST Steak and Sunny-Side Up Eggs with Skillet Tomatoes
SNACK Quinoa-Sesame Buckwheat Crackers
LUNCH Avocado-Basil Chicken Salad
SNACK Cayenne-Spiced Walnuts
DINNER Lemony Pot Roast
DESSERT Chai-Coconut Ice Pops

Day 13

BREAKFAST Coconut-Almond Waffles
SNACK Cayenne-Spiced Walnuts
LUNCH Almond Butter Bread
SNACK Trail Mix
DINNER Poached Salmon with Warm Tomatoes
DESSERT I Scream for Vanilla Ice Cream

Day 14

BREAKFAST Poached Eggs with Quinoa and Spinach
SNACK Oven-Roasted Onion-Garlic Dip
LUNCH Poached Salmon and Avocado Salad
SNACK Roasted Radicchio with Thyme
DINNER Poached Salmon with Warm Tomatoes
DESSERT Chocolate "Milkshake"

Day 15

BREAKFAST Zucchini-Herb Frittata
SNACK Spicy Baked Chicken Wings
LUNCH Grilled Skirt Steak Arugula Salad with Cilantro-Lime Vinaigrette
SNACK Chili-Lime Jicama with Diced Cucumbers
DINNER Grilled Moroccan Salmon
DESSERT Nutty Coconut Bark

Day 16

BREAKFAST Poached Eggs with Quinoa and Spinach
SNACK Puffed Quinoa Treats
LUNCH Grilled Chicken and Arugula Salad
SNACK Quinoa with Fresh Herb Vinaigrette
DINNER Pan-Seared Herring with Lime and Pepper
DESSERT Fresh Mint Bars

Day 17

BREAKFAST Baked Eggs with Kale and Yogurt
SNACK Chili-Lime Jicama with Diced Cucumbers
LUNCH Classic Egg Drop Soup
SNACK Garlicky Mixed Bitter Greens
DINNER Slow-Roasted Lamb Shoulder with Lemons
DESSERT Chai-Coconut Ice Pops

Day 18

BREAKFAST Steak and Sunny-Side Up
Eggs with Skillet Tomatoes
SNACK Spicy Baked Chicken Wings
LUNCH Spinach-Celeriac Soup
SNACK Trail Mix
DINNER Lamb Vindaloo
DESSERT I Scream for Vanilla
Ice Cream

Day 19

BREAKFAST Coconut-Almond Waffles
SNACK Gingery Brussels Sprouts
LUNCH Avocado-Basil Chicken Salad
SNACK Roasted Radicchio with Thyme
DINNER Vegetable "Fried Rice"
DESSERT Chocolate "Milkshake"

Day 20

BREAKFAST Poached Eggs with Quinoa
and Spinach
SNACK Garlicky Mixed Bitter Greens
LUNCH Almond Butter Bread
SNACK Cayenne-Spiced Walnuts
DINNER Lime-Garlic Chicken with
Avocado Salsa
DESSERT Nutty Coconut Bark

Day 21

BREAKFAST Zucchini-Herb Frittata
SNACK Gingery Brussels Sprouts
LUNCH Cream of Roasted
Cauliflower Soup
SNACK Puffed Quinoa Treats
DINNER Kid-Friendly Chicken Fingers
DESSERT Fresh Mint Bars

Day 22

BREAKFAST Poached Eggs with Quinoa
and Spinach
SNACK Chili-Lime Jicama with Diced
Cucumbers
LUNCH Kale Salad with Toasted
Walnuts and Eggs
SNACK Quinoa-Sesame Buckwheat
Crackers
DINNER Grilled Beef Skewers with
Zucchini
DESSERT Chai-Coconut Ice Pops

Day 23

BREAKFAST Baked Eggs with Kale
and Yogurt
SNACK Quinoa-Sesame Buckwheat
Crackers
LUNCH Grilled Skirt Steak Arugula
Salad with Cilantro-Lime Vinaigrette
SNACK Spicy Baked Chicken Wings
DINNER Salmon with Garlic and Ginger
DESSERT I Scream for Vanilla
Ice Cream

Day 24

BREAKFAST Steak and Sunny-Side Up Eggs with Skillet Tomatoes
SNACK Cayenne-Spiced Walnuts
LUNCH Grilled Chicken and Arugula Salad
SNACK Trail Mix
DINNER Garlic and Rosemary Chicken Thighs
DESSERT Chocolate "Milkshake"

Day 25

BREAKFAST Coconut-Almond Waffles
SNACK Quinoa-Sesame Buckwheat Crackers
LUNCH Almond Butter Bread
SNACK Oven-Roasted Onion-Garlic Dip
DINNER Vegetable "Fried Rice"
DESSERT Fresh Mint Bars

Day 26

BREAKFAST Poached Eggs with Quinoa and Spinach
SNACK Cayenne-Spiced Walnuts
LUNCH Kale Salad with Toasted Walnuts and Eggs
SNACK Trail Mix
DINNER Lime-Garlic Chicken with Avocado Salsa
DESSERT Chai-Coconut Ice Pops

Day 27

BREAKFAST Zucchini-Herb Frittata
SNACK Oven-Roasted Onion-Garlic Dip
LUNCH Avocado-Basil Chicken Salad
SNACK Roasted Radicchio with Thyme
DINNER Kid-Friendly Chicken Fingers
DESSERT I Scream for Vanilla Ice Cream

Day 28

BREAKFAST Poached Eggs with Quinoa and Spinach
SNACK Spicy Baked Chicken Wings
LUNCH Spinach-Celeriac Soup
SNACK Chili-Lime Jicama with Diced Cucumbers
DINNER Grilled Beef Skewers with Zucchini
DESSERT Chocolate "Milkshake"

Day 29

BREAKFAST Baked Eggs with Kale and Yogurt
SNACK Puffed Quinoa Treats
LUNCH Grilled Chicken and Arugula Salad
SNACK Quinoa with Fresh Herb Vinaigrette
DINNER Salmon with Garlic and Ginger
DESSERT Nutty Coconut Bark

Day 30

BREAKFAST Steak and Sunny-Side Up Eggs with Skillet Tomatoes
SNACK Chili-Lime Jicama with Diced Cucumbers
LUNCH Classic Egg Drop Soup
SNACK Garlicky Mixed Bitter Greens
DINNER Grilled Sirloin with Garlic Butter
DESSERT Fresh Mint Bars

Day 31

BREAKFAST Coconut-Almond Waffles
SNACK Trail Mix
LUNCH Grilled Skirt Steak Arugula Salad with Cilantro-Lime Vinaigrette
SNACK Oven-Roasted Onion-Garlic Dip
DINNER Garlic and Rosemary Chicken Thighs
DESSERT Chai-Coconut Ice Pops

Day 32

BREAKFAST Poached Eggs with Quinoa and Spinach
SNACK Gingery Brussels Sprouts
LUNCH Poached Salmon and Avocado Salad
SNACK Spicy Baked Chicken Wings
DINNER Lentil Curry with Spinach
DESSERT I Scream for Vanilla Ice Cream

Day 33

BREAKFAST Zucchini-Herb Frittata
SNACK Garlicky Mixed Bitter Greens
LUNCH Cream of Roasted Cauliflower Soup
SNACK Puffed Quinoa Treats
DINNER Coconut Chicken with Bok Choy
DESSERT Chocolate "Milkshake"

Day 34

BREAKFAST Poached Eggs with Quinoa and Spinach
SNACK Roasted Radicchio with Thyme
LUNCH Tomato Florentine Soup
SNACK Gingery Brussels Sprouts
DINNER Spicy Chicken Patties
DESSERT Nutty Coconut Bark

Day 35

BREAKFAST Baked Eggs with Kale and Yogurt
SNACK Quinoa with Fresh Herb Vinaigrette
LUNCH Kale Salad with Toasted Walnuts and Eggs
SNACK Quinoa-Sesame Buckwheat Crackers
DINNER Herb-Roasted Turkey Tenderloin
DESSERT Fresh Mint Bars

Day 36

BREAKFAST Steak and Sunny-Side Up Eggs with Skillet Tomatoes
SNACK Quinoa-Sesame Buckwheat Crackers
LUNCH Avocado-Basil Chicken Salad
SNACK Cayenne-Spiced Walnuts
DINNER Lemony Pot Roast
DESSERT Chai-Coconut Ice Pops

Day 37

BREAKFAST Coconut-Almond Waffles
SNACK Cayenne-Spiced Walnuts
LUNCH Almond Butter Bread
SNACK Trail Mix
DINNER Poached Salmon with Warm Tomatoes
DESSERT I Scream for Vanilla Ice Cream

Day 38

BREAKFAST Poached Eggs with Quinoa and Spinach
SNACK Oven-Roasted Onion-Garlic Dip
LUNCH Poached Salmon and Avocado Salad
SNACK Roasted Radicchio with Thyme
DINNER Poached Salmon with Warm Tomatoes
DESSERT Chocolate "Milkshake"

Day 39

BREAKFAST Zucchini-Herb Frittata
SNACK Spicy Baked Chicken Wings
LUNCH Grilled Skirt Steak Arugula Salad with Cilantro-Lime Vinaigrette
SNACK Chili-Lime Jicama with Diced Cucumbers
DINNER Grilled Moroccan Salmon
DESSERT Nutty Coconut Bark

Day 40

BREAKFAST Poached Eggs with Quinoa and Spinach
SNACK Puffed Quinoa Treats
LUNCH Grilled Chicken and Arugula Salad
SNACK Quinoa with Fresh Herb Vinaigrette
DINNER Pan-Seared Herring with Lime and Pepper
DESSERT Fresh Mint Bars

Day 41

BREAKFAST Baked Eggs with Kale and Yogurt
SNACK Chili-Lime Jicama with Diced Cucumbers
LUNCH Classic Egg Drop Soup
SNACK Garlicky Mixed Bitter Greens
DINNER Slow-Roasted Lamb Shoulder with Lemons
DESSERT Chai-Coconut Ice Pops

Day 42

BREAKFAST Steak and Sunny-Side Up Eggs with Skillet Tomatoes
SNACK Spicy Baked Chicken Wings
LUNCH Spinach-Celeriac Soup
SNACK Trail Mix
DINNER Lamb Vindaloo
DESSERT I Scream for Vanilla Ice Cream

Day 43

BREAKFAST Coconut-Almond Waffles
SNACK Gingery Brussels Sprouts
LUNCH Avocado-Basil Chicken Salad
SNACK Roasted Radicchio with Thyme
DINNER Vegetable "Fried Rice"
DESSERT Chocolate "Milkshake"

Day 44

BREAKFAST Poached Eggs with Quinoa and Spinach
SNACK Garlicky Mixed Bitter Greens
LUNCH Almond Butter Bread
SNACK Spicy Baked Chicken Wings
DINNER Lime-Garlic Chicken with Avocado Salsa
DESSERT Nutty Coconut Bark

Day 45

BREAKFAST Zucchini-Herb Frittata
SNACK Gingery Brussels Sprouts
LUNCH Cream of Roasted Cauliflower Soup
SNACK Puffed Quinoa Treats
DINNER Kid-Friendly Chicken Fingers
DESSERT Fresh Mint Bars

Day 46

BREAKFAST Poached Eggs with Quinoa and Spinach
SNACK Chili-Lime Jicama with Diced Cucumbers
LUNCH Kale Salad with Toasted Walnuts and Eggs
SNACK Quinoa-Sesame Buckwheat Crackers
DINNER Grilled Beef Skewers with Zucchini
DESSERT Chai-Coconut Ice Pops

Day 47

BREAKFAST Baked Eggs with Kale and Yogurt
SNACK Quinoa-Sesame Buckwheat Crackers
LUNCH Grilled Skirt Steak Arugula Salad with Cilantro-Lime Vinaigrette
SNACK Spicy Baked Chicken Wings
DINNER Salmon with Garlic and Ginger
DESSERT I Scream for Vanilla Ice Cream

Day 48

BREAKFAST Steak and Sunny-Side Up Eggs with Skillet Tomatoes
SNACK Cayenne-Spiced Walnuts
LUNCH Grilled Chicken and Arugula Salad
SNACK Trail Mix
DINNER Garlic and Rosemary Chicken Thighs
DESSERT Chocolate "Milkshake"

Day 49

BREAKFAST Coconut-Almond Waffles
SNACK Quinoa-Sesame Buckwheat Crackers
LUNCH Almond Butter Bread
SNACK Oven-Roasted Onion-Garlic Dip
DINNER Vegetable "Fried Rice"
DESSERT Fresh Mint Bars

Day 50

BREAKFAST Poached Eggs with Quinoa and Spinach
SNACK Cayenne-Spiced Walnuts
LUNCH Kale Salad with Toasted Walnuts and Eggs
SNACK Trail Mix
DINNER Lime-Garlic Chicken with Avocado Salsa
DESSERT Chai-Coconut Ice Pops

Day 51

BREAKFAST Zucchini-Herb Frittata
SNACK Oven-Roasted Onion-Garlic Dip
LUNCH Avocado-Basil Chicken Salad
SNACK Roasted Radicchio with Thyme
DINNER Kid-Friendly Chicken Fingers
DESSERT I Scream for Vanilla Ice Cream

Day 52

BREAKFAST Poached Eggs with Quinoa and Spinach
SNACK Spicy Baked Chicken Wings
LUNCH Spinach-Celeriac Soup
SNACK Chili-Lime Jicama with Diced Cucumbers
DINNER Grilled Beef Skewers with Zucchini
DESSERT Chocolate "Milkshake"

Day 53

BREAKFAST Baked Eggs with Kale and Yogurt
SNACK Puffed Quinoa Treats
LUNCH Grilled Chicken and Arugula Salad
SNACK Quinoa with Fresh Herb Vinaigrette
DINNER Salmon with Garlic and Ginger
DESSERT Nutty Coconut Bark

Day 54

BREAKFAST Steak and Sunny-Side Up Eggs with Skillet Tomatoes
SNACK Chili-Lime Jicama with Diced Cucumbers
LUNCH Classic Egg Drop Soup
SNACK Garlicky Mixed Bitter Greens
DINNER Grilled Sirloin with Garlic Butter
DESSERT Fresh Mint Bars

Day 55

BREAKFAST Coconut-Almond Waffles
SNACK Trail Mix
LUNCH Grilled Skirt Steak Arugula Salad with Cilantro-Lime Vinaigrette
SNACK Oven-Roasted Onion-Garlic Dip
DINNER Garlic and Rosemary Chicken Thighs
DESSERT Chai-Coconut Ice Pops

Day 56

BREAKFAST Poached Eggs with Quinoa and Spinach
SNACK Gingery Brussels Sprouts
LUNCH Poached Salmon and Avocado Salad
SNACK Spicy Baked Chicken Wings
DINNER Lentil Curry with Spinach
DESSERT I Scream for Vanilla Ice Cream

Day 57

BREAKFAST Zucchini-Herb Frittata
SNACK Garlicky Mixed Bitter Greens
LUNCH Cream of Roasted Cauliflower Soup
SNACK Puffed Quinoa Treats
DINNER Coconut Chicken with Bok Choy
DESSERT Chocolate "Milkshake"

Day 58

BREAKFAST Poached Eggs with Quinoa and Spinach
SNACK Roasted Radicchio with Thyme
LUNCH Tomato Florentine Soup
SNACK Gingery Brussels Sprouts
DINNER Spicy Chicken Patties
DESSERT Nutty Coconut Bark

Day 59

BREAKFAST Baked Eggs with Kale and Yogurt
SNACK Quinoa with Fresh Herb Vinaigrette
LUNCH Kale Salad with Toasted Walnuts and Eggs
SNACK Quinoa-Sesame Buckwheat Crackers
DINNER Herb-Roasted Turkey Tenderloin
DESSERT Fresh Mint Bars

Day 60

BREAKFAST Steak and Sunny-Side Up Eggs with Skillet Tomatoes
SNACK Quinoa-Sesame Buckwheat Crackers
LUNCH Avocado-Basil Chicken Salad
SNACK Cayenne-Spiced Walnuts
DINNER Lemony Pot Roast
DESSERT Chai-Coconut Ice Pops

Day 61

BREAKFAST Coconut-Almond Waffles
SNACK Cayenne-Spiced Walnuts
LUNCH Almond Butter Bread
SNACK Trail Mix
DINNER Poached Salmon with Warm Tomatoes
DESSERT I Scream for Vanilla Ice Cream

Day 62

BREAKFAST Poached Eggs with Quinoa and Spinach
SNACK Oven-Roasted Onion-Garlic Dip
LUNCH Poached Salmon and Avocado Salad
SNACK Roasted Radicchio with Thyme
DINNER Poached Salmon with Warm Tomatoes
DESSERT Chocolate "Milkshake"

Day 63

BREAKFAST Zucchini-Herb Frittata
SNACK Spicy Baked Chicken Wings
LUNCH Grilled Skirt Steak Arugula Salad with Cilantro-Lime Vinaigrette
SNACK Chili-Lime Jicama with Diced Cucumbers
DINNER Grilled Moroccan Salmon
DESSERT Nutty Coconut Bark

Day 64

BREAKFAST Poached Eggs with Quinoa and Spinach
SNACK Puffed Quinoa Treats
LUNCH Grilled Chicken and Arugula Salad
SNACK Quinoa with Fresh Herb Vinaigrette
DINNER Pan-Seared Herring with Lime and Pepper
DESSERT Fresh Mint Bars

Day 65

BREAKFAST Baked Eggs with Kale and Yogurt
SNACK Chili-Lime Jicama with Diced Cucumbers
LUNCH Classic Egg Drop Soup
SNACK Garlicky Mixed Bitter Greens
DINNER Slow-Roasted Lamb Shoulder with Lemons
DESSERT Chai-Coconut Ice Pops

Day 66

BREAKFAST Steak and Sunny-Side Up Eggs with Skillet Tomatoes
SNACK Spicy Baked Chicken Wings
LUNCH Spinach-Celeriac Soup
SNACK Trail Mix
DINNER Lamb Vindaloo
DESSERT I Scream for Vanilla Ice Cream

Day 67

BREAKFAST Coconut-Almond Waffles
SNACK Gingery Brussels Sprouts
LUNCH Avocado-Basil Chicken Salad
SNACK Roasted Radicchio with Thyme
DINNER Vegetable "Fried Rice"
DESSERT Chocolate "Milkshake"

Day 68

BREAKFAST Poached Eggs with Quinoa and Spinach
SNACK Garlicky Mixed Bitter Greens
LUNCH Almond Butter Bread
SNACK Roasted Radicchio with Thyme
DINNER Lime-Garlic Chicken with Avocado Salsa
DESSERT Nutty Coconut Bark

Day 69

BREAKFAST Zucchini-Herb Frittata
SNACK Gingery Brussels Sprouts
LUNCH Cream of Roasted Cauliflower Soup
SNACK Puffed Quinoa Treats
DINNER Kid-Friendly Chicken Fingers
DESSERT Fresh Mint Bars

Day 70

BREAKFAST Poached Eggs with Quinoa and Spinach
SNACK Chili-Lime Jicama with Diced Cucumbers
LUNCH Kale Salad with Toasted Walnuts and Eggs
SNACK Quinoa-Sesame Buckwheat Crackers
DINNER Grilled Beef Skewers with Zucchini
DESSERT Chai-Coconut Ice Pops

Day 71

BREAKFAST Baked Eggs with Kale and Yogurt
SNACK Quinoa-Sesame Buckwheat Crackers
LUNCH Grilled Skirt Steak Arugula Salad with Cilantro-Lime Vinaigrette
SNACK Spicy Baked Chicken Wings
DINNER Salmon with Garlic and Ginger
DESSERT I Scream for Vanilla Ice Cream

Day 72

BREAKFAST Steak and Sunny-Side Up Eggs with Skillet Tomatoes
SNACK Cayenne-Spiced Walnuts
LUNCH Grilled Chicken and Arugula Salad
SNACK Trail Mix
DINNER Garlic and Rosemary Chicken Thighs
DESSERT Chocolate "Milkshake"

Day 73

BREAKFAST Zucchini-Herb Frittata
SNACK Gingery Brussels Sprouts
LUNCH Cream of Roasted
Cauliflower Soup
SNACK Puffed Quinoa Treats
DINNER Kid-Friendly Chicken Fingers
DESSERT Fresh Mint Bars

Day 74

BREAKFAST Poached Eggs with Quinoa
and Spinach
SNACK Chili-Lime Jicama with
Diced Cucumbers
LUNCH Kale Salad with Toasted
Walnuts and Eggs
SNACK Quinoa-Sesame
Buckwheat Crackers
DINNER Grilled Beef Skewers with
Zucchini
DESSERT Chai-Coconut Ice Pops

Day 75

BREAKFAST Baked Eggs with Kale and
Yogurt
SNACK Quinoa-Sesame Buckwheat
Crackers
LUNCH Grilled Skirt Steak Arugula
Salad with Cilantro-Lime Vinaigrette
SNACK Spicy Baked Chicken Wings
DINNER Salmon with Garlic and Ginger
DESSERT I Scream for Vanilla
Ice Cream

Day 76

BREAKFAST Steak and Sunny-Side Up
Eggs with Skillet Tomatoes
SNACK Cayenne-Spiced Walnuts
LUNCH Grilled Chicken and
Arugula Salad
SNACK Trail Mix
DINNER Garlic and Rosemary
Chicken Thighs
DESSERT Chocolate "Milkshake"

Day 77

*Transition to Maintenance
Mode Begins*

BREAKFAST Coconut-Almond Waffles
SNACK Berry Skewers with
Chia-Yogurt Dip
LUNCH Beef and Vegetable Stew
SNACK Quinoa-Sesame Buckwheat
Crackers
DINNER Salmon with Garlic and Ginger
DESSERT Warm Apple Bake with
Streusel Topping

Day 78

BREAKFAST Sweetie Pie Smoothie
SNACK Roasted Beet and Garlic
"Hummus"
LUNCH Chicken and Sweet Potato Soup
with Collard Greens
SNACK Spicy Baked Chicken Wings
DINNER Grilled Beef Skewers with
Zucchini
DESSERT I Scream for Vanilla
Ice Cream

Day 79

BREAKFAST Quinoa Porridge with Cardamom, Almonds, and Sliced Pear
SNACK Roasted Ginger-Cumin Chickpeas
LUNCH Kale Salad with Toasted Walnuts and Eggs
SNACK Puffed Quinoa Treats
DINNER Roasted Chicken with Pears
DESSERT Almond-Chocolate Truffles

Day 80

BREAKFAST Strawberry Muffins
SNACK Savory and Sweet Potato Chips
LUNCH Ground Lamb and Lentil Lettuce Wraps
SNACK Chili-Lime Jicama with Diced Cucumbers
DINNER Grilled Sirloin with Garlic Butter
DESSERT Nutty Coconut Bark

Day 81

BREAKFAST Zucchini-Herb Frittata
SNACK Berry Savory Ants on a Log
LUNCH Mexican-Spiced Tomato and White Bean Soup
SNACK Mashed Parsnips and Apples
DINNER Herbed Chicken with White Beans
DESSERT Mixed-Berry Slushie

Day 82

BREAKFAST Coconut Millet with Cacao and Raspberries
SNACK Roasted Eggplant Tapenade
LUNCH Grilled Chicken and Arugula Salad
SNACK Coconut-Lime Sweet Potatoes
DINNER Lemony Pot Roast
DESSERT Chocolate "Milkshake"

Day 83

BREAKFAST Blueberry-Lemon Pancakes
SNACK Carrots with Gremolata
LUNCH Quinoa Salad with Roasted Sweet Potato and Apples
SNACK Roasted Radicchio with Thyme
DINNER Turkey Cabbage Rolls
DESSERT Strawberry Shortcake

Day 84

BREAKFAST Coconut-Almond Waffles
SNACK Berry Skewers with Chia-Yogurt Dip
LUNCH Beef and Vegetable Stew
SNACK Quinoa-Sesame Buckwheat Crackers
DINNER Salmon with Garlic and Ginger
DESSERT Warm Apple Bake with Streusel Topping

Day 85

BREAKFAST Sweetie Pie Smoothie
SNACK Roasted Beet and Garlic "Hummus"
LUNCH Chicken and Sweet Potato Soup with Collard Greens
SNACK Spicy Baked Chicken Wings
DINNER Grilled Beef Skewers with Zucchini
DESSERT I Scream for Vanilla Ice Cream

Day 86

BREAKFAST Quinoa Porridge with Cardamom, Almonds, and Sliced Pear
SNACK Roasted Ginger-Cumin Chickpeas
LUNCH Kale Salad with Toasted Walnuts and Eggs
SNACK Puffed Quinoa Treats
DINNER Roasted Chicken with Pears
DESSERT Almond-Chocolate Truffles

Day 87

BREAKFAST Strawberry Muffins
SNACK Savory and Sweet Potato Chips
LUNCH Ground Lamb and Lentil Lettuce Wraps
SNACK Chili-Lime Jicama with Diced Cucumbers
DINNER Grilled Sirloin with Garlic Butter
DESSERT Nutty Coconut Bark

Day 88

BREAKFAST Zucchini-Herb Frittata
SNACK Berry Savory Ants on a Log
LUNCH Mexican-Spiced Tomato and White Bean Soup
SNACK Mashed Parsnips and Apples
DINNER Herbed Chicken with White Beans
DESSERT Mixed-Berry Slushie

Day 89

BREAKFAST Coconut Millet with Cacao and Raspberries
SNACK Roasted Eggplant Tapenade
LUNCH Grilled Chicken and Arugula Salad
SNACK Coconut-Lime Sweet Potatoes
DINNER Lemony Pot Roast
DESSERT Chocolate "Milkshake"

Day 90

BREAKFAST Blueberry-Lemon Pancakes
SNACK Carrots with Gremolata
LUNCH Quinoa Salad with Roasted Sweet Potato and Apples
SNACK Roasted Radicchio with Thyme
DINNER Turkey Cabbage Rolls
DESSERT Strawberry Shortcake

Seven-Day Maintenance Mode Meal Plan

Day 1

BREAKFAST Coconut-Almond Waffles
SNACK Berry Skewers with
Chia-Yogurt Dip
LUNCH Beef and Vegetable Stew
SNACK Quinoa-Sesame Buckwheat
Crackers
DINNER Salmon with Garlic and Ginger
DESSERT Warm Apple Bake with
Streusel Topping

Day 2

BREAKFAST Sweetie Pie Smoothie
SNACK Roasted Beet and Garlic
"Hummus"
LUNCH Chicken and Sweet Potato Soup
with Collard Greens
SNACK Spicy Baked Chicken Wings
DINNER Grilled Beef Skewers with
Zucchini
DESSERT I Scream for Vanilla
Ice Cream

Day 3

BREAKFAST Quinoa Porridge with
Cardamom, Almonds, and Sliced Pear
SNACK Roasted Ginger-Cumin
Chickpeas
LUNCH Kale Salad with Toasted
Walnuts and Eggs
SNACK Puffed Quinoa Treats
DINNER Roasted Chicken with Pears
DESSERT Almond-Chocolate Truffles

Day 4

BREAKFAST Strawberry Muffins
SNACK Savory and Sweet Potato Chips
LUNCH Ground Lamb and Lentil
Lettuce Wraps
SNACK Chili-Lime Jicama with Diced
Cucumbers
DINNER Grilled Sirloin with
Garlic Butter
DESSERT Nutty Coconut Bark

Day 5

BREAKFAST Zucchini-Herb Frittata
SNACK Berry Savory Ants on a Log
LUNCH Mexican-Spiced Tomato and
White Bean Soup
SNACK Mashed Parsnips and Apples
DINNER Herbed Chicken with
White Beans
DESSERT Mixed-Berry Slushie

Day 6

BREAKFAST Coconut Millet with Cacao and Raspberries
SNACK Roasted Eggplant Tapenade
LUNCH Grilled Chicken and Arugula Salad
SNACK Coconut-Lime Sweet Potatoes
DINNER Lemony Pot Roast
DESSERT Chocolate "Milkshake"

Day 7

BREAKFAST Blueberry-Lemon Pancakes
SNACK Carrots with Gremolata
LUNCH Quinoa Salad with Roasted Sweet Potato and Apples
SNACK Roasted Radicchio with Thyme
DINNER Turkey Cabbage Rolls
DESSERT Strawberry Shortcake

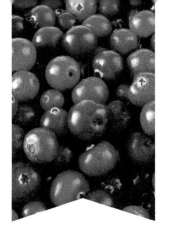

PART II

Candida Diet Recipes

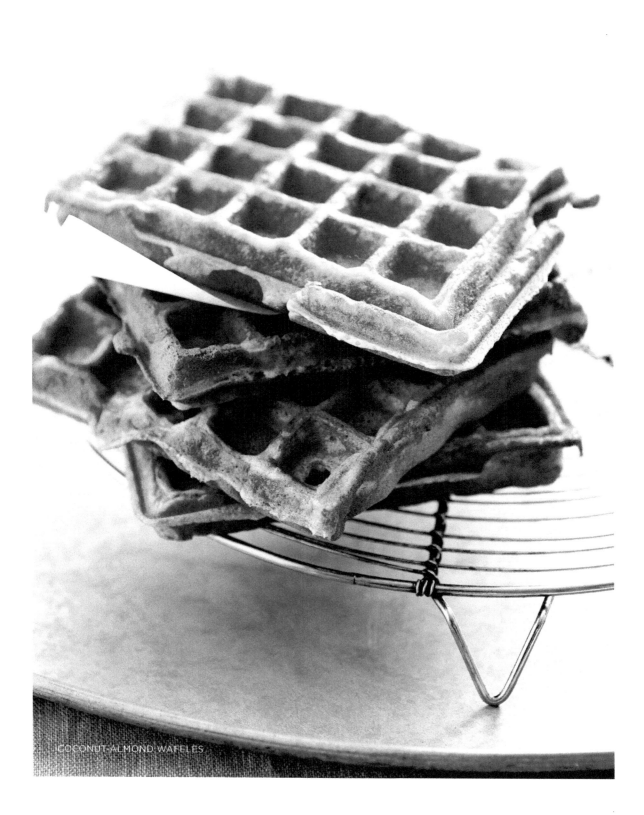

COCONUT-ALMOND WAFFLES

5

Breakfasts

CLEANSE

PECAN-BUCKWHEAT PORRIDGE

COCONUT-ALMOND WAFFLES

HERBED AVOCADO OMELET

ZUCCHINI-HERB FRITTATA

POACHED EGGS WITH QUINOA AND SPINACH

BAKED EGGS WITH KALE AND YOGURT

TASTY EGG MUFFINS

STEAK AND SUNNY-SIDE UP EGGS WITH SKILLET TOMATOES

MAINTENANCE

QUINOA PORRIDGE WITH CARDAMOM, ALMONDS, AND SLICED PEAR

SWEETIE PIE SMOOTHIE

STRAWBERRY MUFFINS

BLUEBERRY-LEMON PANCAKES

COCONUT MILLET WITH CACAO AND RASPBERRIES

COCONUT CUSTARD WITH PINEAPPLE

VERY BERRY PARFAIT

Pecan-Buckwheat Porridge

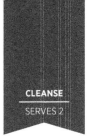

This nutrient-packed hot cereal might take a little bit of time to get used to, especially if you are used to packaged instant oatmeal. Buckwheat has an assertive flavor that is almost nutty, so it combines well with the almond milk. If you prefer, you can use unsweetened coconut milk instead of almond milk.

2 CUPS WATER

½ CUP BUCKWHEAT

½ CUP OAT BRAN

1 CUP UNSWEETENED ALMOND MILK

¼ TEASPOON GROUND CINNAMON

PINCH STEVIA

2 TABLESPOONS CHOPPED PECANS

1. Place the water in a large saucepan over medium-high heat and bring it to a boil.

2. Add the buckwheat and boil it until the buckwheat expands, about 15 minutes.

3. Stir in the oat bran and reduce the heat to low. Continue to cook the mixture until the water is absorbed, about 10 minutes.

4. Remove the saucepan from heat and let the mixture stand for 5 minutes.

5. Stir in the almond milk, cinnamon, stevia, and pecans and serve warm.

CALORIES: 403   TOTAL FAT: 16 G   SATURATED FAT: 2 G   SUGAR: 5 G   CARBOHYDRATES: 57 G
NUTRITIONAL VALUE IS PER SERVING UNLESS OTHERWISE SPECIFIED.

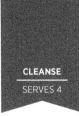

Coconut-Almond Waffles

You may be watching what you eat, but you can still make breakfast for friends and family. A crowd pleaser, this recipe may be topped off with a dollop of probiotic yogurt and a sprinkle of unsweetened shredded coconut, and still remain candida-free. Carry this dish through to your maintenance phase, when you can sweeten it up with mixed berries. If you don't have a waffle iron, just use this same batter to make pancakes.

2 EGGS

1 CUP UNSWEETENED COCONUT MILK

1 CUP SHREDDED UNSWEETENED
    COCONUT

½ CUP ALMOND FLOUR

½ TEASPOON SEA SALT

½ TEASPOON GLUTEN-FREE
    BAKING POWDER

½ TEASPOON CINNAMON

NONSTICK COOKING SPRAY

1. In a large mixing bowl, whisk together the eggs and coconut milk. Stir in the shredded coconut, almond flour, salt, baking powder, and cinnamon.

2. Heat a waffle iron and spray it with cooking spray. Pour the batter onto the waffle iron and the close lid. Cook the waffle for 2 to 3 minutes, until the waffle is light brown and crispy.

3. Repeat until all the batter is used up. Serve 2 waffles per plate.

———————

CALORIES: 262   TOTAL FAT: 26 G   SATURATED FAT: 20 G   SUGAR: 4 G   CARBOHYDRATES: 8 G

Herbed Avocado Omelet

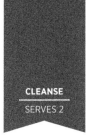
You might find yourself craving this unique, fragrant omelet for lunch or dinner as well as in the morning. The combination of onion and garlic packs a powerful anti-candida punch because they are antifungals and help detox the body. Try any combination of fresh herbs to suit your palate.

6 EGGS, BEATEN

1 TABLESPOON CHOPPED
    FRESH THYME

1 TABLESPOON CHOPPED
    FRESH PARSLEY

1 TOMATO, DICED

2 TEASPOONS BUTTER

¼ SWEET ONION, PEELED AND
    FINELY DICED

1 TEASPOON MINCED GARLIC

1 AVOCADO, PEELED, PITTED,
    AND SLICED

SEA SALT

FRESHLY GROUND BLACK PEPPER

1. In a medium bowl, combine the eggs, thyme, parsley, and tomato, stirring to combine. Set aside.

2. Place a large nonstick skillet on medium-high heat and melt the butter, swirling the pan to coat.

3. Sauté the onion and garlic until they are softened, about 3 minutes.

4. Pour the egg mixture into the pan and stir gently with a heat-proof spatula or wooden spoon. As the egg begins to set, lift the edges and push them slightly toward the center, allowing the uncooked egg to flow underneath.

5. Continue this process until the eggs are completely cooked and fluffy, 2 to 3 minutes.

6. Layer the avocado slices on one half of the omelet. Fold the other half of the omelet over the avocado to create a half moon. Cut the omelet in half and slide the halves onto 2 plates.

7. Season the omelets with salt and pepper and serve warm.

CALORIES: 449 TOTAL FAT: 37 G SATURATED FAT: 11 G SUGAR: 4 G CARBOHYDRATES: 14 G

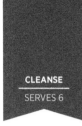

Zucchini-Herb Frittata

If you needed a reason to head to your local farmers' market, preparing this frittata is a great excuse. Treat yourself to the freshest herbs and produce available, and your dish will get an added boost of flavor in the process.

8 EGGS
½ TEASPOON SEA SALT
FRESHLY GROUND BLACK PEPPER
1 TABLESPOON CHOPPED
    FRESH THYME
1 TABLESPOON FINELY CHOPPED
    FRESH PARSLEY

2 TABLESPOONS OLIVE OIL
1 YELLOW ONION, COARSELY CHOPPED
1 ZUCCHINI, CUT IN HALF LENGTHWISE
    AND CUT INTO ¼-INCH SLICES
1 CUP CHOPPED TOMATOES

1. Preheat the broiler.

2. In a medium mixing bowl, whisk together the eggs, salt, pepper, thyme, and parsley. Set aside.

3. Using a large sauté pan, heat the olive oil over medium heat. Sauté the onions and zucchini for 6 minutes, or until they are tender.

4. Stir the tomatoes into the sauté pan and simmer for 2 minutes.

5. Pour in the egg mixture and stir until well combined.

6. Reduce the heat to low and cover. Cook for about 12 minutes, or until the eggs are barely set.

7. Finish the eggs under the broiler for 2 minutes, until they are lightly browned.

8. Remove the frittata from the heat, let it cool slightly, and cut it into wedges to serve.

CALORIES: 160   TOTAL FAT: 11 G   SATURATED FAT: 3 G   SUGAR: 1 G   CARBOHYDRATES: 6 G

Poached Eggs with Quinoa and Spinach

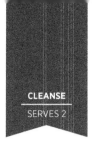

It's true that breakfast is the most important meal of the day. There is no better way to honor it than by starting off your morning with vitamin-packed spinach and protein-rich quinoa. This recipe calls for one cup of cooked quinoa—which you make using just one-quarter cup of uncooked quinoa. For instructions on how to cook quinoa, see the recipe for Quinoa-Sesame Buckwheat Crackers (page 98).

3 TABLESPOONS OLIVE OIL

1 GARLIC CLOVE, SLICED

5 OUNCES BABY SPINACH, RINSED

SEA SALT

1 CARROT, PEELED AND JULIENNED

2 EGGS

1 TEASPOON APPLE CIDER VINEGAR

1 CUP COOKED QUINOA

¼ CUCUMBER, THINLY SLICED

1 TEASPOON MINCED CHIVES

CRUSHED RED PEPPER FLAKES

1. In a large skillet, heat 1 tablespoon of olive oil over medium heat. Add the garlic and cook for 1 minute.

2. Stir in the spinach and cover. Cook for 1 minute more, until the spinach is wilted. Season the garlic-spinach mixture with salt and remove it from the skillet.

3. In a small saucepan, bring 2 inches of water to a boil. Add the carrot and cook for 1 minute, until it's tender. Using a slotted spoon, transfer the carrot to a plate.

4. Reduce the heat to simmer and poach the eggs separately, cooking each for 3 to 4 minutes, or until set. Remove the eggs carefully with a slotted spoon.

5. In a small bowl, whisk together the vinegar and remaining 2 tablespoons of olive oil, then season with salt.

6. Divide the quinoa between 2 bowls. Top each with an egg, spinach, carrot, cucumber, and a drizzle of the vinaigrette. Sprinkle each with chives and a pinch of red pepper flakes.

CALORIES: 367   TOTAL FAT: 27 G   SATURATED FAT: 5 G   SUGAR: 3 G   CARBOHYDRATES: 20 G

Baked Eggs with Kale and Yogurt

Between the creamy dollop of garlic yogurt and the zesty kick of crushed red pepper, these "green" eggs are so good you won't even miss the ham. The recipe calls for you to bake the eggs in one large skillet; if you don't have one, feel free to divide the recipe and cook it in two smaller skillets.

⅔ CUP PLAIN GREEK YOGURT

1 GARLIC CLOVE, HALVED

SEA SALT

2 TABLESPOONS UNSALTED BUTTER

2 TABLESPOONS OLIVE OIL

3 TABLESPOONS CHOPPED LEEK, WHITE AND LIGHT-GREEN PARTS

2 TABLESPOONS CHOPPED SCALLIONS, WHITE AND LIGHT-GREEN PARTS

10 OUNCES TUSCAN KALE, CENTER RIBS DISCARDED, COARSELY CHOPPED

1 TEASPOON FRESHLY SQUEEZED LEMON JUICE

4 EGGS

¼ TEASPOON CRUSHED RED PEPPER

PINCH PAPRIKA

1 TEASPOON CHOPPED FRESH OREGANO

1. Preheat the oven to 300°F.

2. In a small mixing bowl, combine the yogurt, garlic, and a pinch of salt. Set aside.

3. In a large sauté pan or skillet, melt 1 tablespoon of butter with the olive oil over medium heat. Stir in the leek and scallions. Reduce the heat to low and cook for about 10 minutes, until they soften.

4. Stir in the kale and lemon juice, and season with salt. Raise the heat to medium-high and cook for 5 minutes, stirring continuously, until kale is wilted.

5. Using a slotted spoon, transfer the kale mixture to a large oven-safe skillet, making an even layer. Hollow out 4 indentations in the kale mixture; break 1 egg into each hollow.

6. Put the skillet in the oven and bake until the eggs have set, 10 to 15 minutes.

7. In a small saucepan, melt the remaining 1 tablespoon of butter over medium-low heat. Whisk in the crushed red pepper and paprika. Cook for 1 to 2 minutes, until the butter starts to foam and brown bits start to form at the bottom of the pan.

8. Stir in the oregano and cook for 30 seconds. Remove the saucepan from the heat.

9. Divide the egg and kale mixture between 4 plates. Remove the garlic from the yogurt and spoon the yogurt over the eggs; discard the garlic. Top off each egg with a drizzle of crushed red pepper butter.

CALORIES: 223   TOTAL FAT: 64 G   SATURATED FAT: 16 G   SUGAR: 3 G   CARBOHYDRATES: 7 G

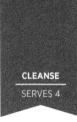

Tasty Egg Muffins

These tempting muffins are the ultimate grab-and-go breakfast, either warm or cold. You can wrap them up individually and store the muffins in the freezer until you want to enjoy one. Simply microwave each egg muffin about 30 seconds to reheat it.

NONSTICK COOKING SPRAY

2 GREEN ONIONS, CHOPPED

2 TEASPOONS MINCED GARLIC

2 TOMATOES, CHOPPED

4 ASPARAGUS SPEARS, CHOPPED

½ CUP SHREDDED SPINACH

2 TABLESPOONS CHOPPED
  FRESH BASIL

8 EGG WHITES

6 EGGS

1. Preheat the oven to 375°F.

2. Spray a 12-cup muffin pan with nonstick cooking spray. Set aside.

3. In a large bowl, toss together the onions, garlic, tomatoes, asparagus, spinach, and basil until well combined.

4. In a medium bowl, beat together the egg whites and whole eggs.

5. Fill the muffin tins evenly with the egg mixture.

6. Scoop the vegetable mixture on top of the eggs, dividing the vegetables evenly. Carefully stir each cup to distribute the vegetables.

7. Bake the muffins for 20 to 30 minutes or until the muffins are firm.

8. Run a knife around the finished muffins and pop them out of the pan.

9. Serve the muffins warm or cold.

CALORIES: 148   TOTAL FAT: 7 G   SATURATED FAT: 2 G   SUGAR: 3 G   CARBOHYDRATES: 6 G

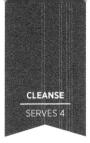
Steak and Sunny-Side Up Eggs with Skillet Tomatoes

Flank steak is full of flavor, it's budget-friendly, it cooks quickly, and it's a relatively lean and low-calorie cut of beef. Teaming it up with eggs and seared tomatoes makes for a classic, hearty dish that may make you even forget that you're on a special diet.

1 TABLESPOON OLIVE OIL,
    PLUS 1 TEASPOON
1 POUND FLANK STEAK
SEA SALT
FRESHLY GROUND BLACK PEPPER

4 TOMATOES, HALVED
NONSTICK COOKING SPRAY
4 EGGS
1 TABLESPOON CHOPPED FRESH
    OREGANO

1. In a large skillet, heat 1 tablespoon of olive oil over medium-high heat.

2. Season the flank steak with salt and pepper. Cook the steak in the skillet for 4 to 5 minutes per side. Remove the steak from the skillet and let it rest for 5 minutes, then slice it against the grain.

3. Add the tomatoes to the same skillet, cut-side down. Cook the tomatoes for 2 to 3 minutes, until browned.

4. While the tomatoes cook, spray another skillet with nonstick cooking spray. Crack the eggs into the skillet and cook 2 to 4 minutes, until perfectly sunny-side up. Remove the eggs from the heat.

5. Divide the steak among 4 plates. Slide 1 egg and half a tomato next to each mound of steak. Top the eggs and tomatoes with oregano, salt, and pepper.

CALORIES: 306   TOTAL FAT: 17 G   SATURATED FAT: 5 G   SUGAR: 4 G   CARBOHYDRATES: 7 G

Quinoa Porridge with Cardamom, Almonds, and Sliced Pear

If you have a taste for the exotic, this spiced hot cereal will tickle your fancy. Popular in Indian cuisine, cardamom will give any ho-hum dish a dash of depth. If you can't find the aromatic spice at your local market, you can substitute a blend of equal parts cinnamon and nutmeg for a similar flavor profile.

½ CUP RINSED UNCOOKED QUINOA

1¾ CUPS UNSWEETENED ALMOND MILK

½ CUP WATER

¼ TEASPOON SEA SALT

¼ TEASPOON GROUND CARDAMOM

STEVIA

1 PEAR, SLICED

4 TABLESPOONS SLICED ALMONDS, TOASTED

1. In a medium saucepan, bring the quinoa, ¾ cup of almond milk, water, salt, and cardamom to a boil. Reduce the heat and simmer, covered, for 15 minutes, until the liquid is absorbed. Remove the quinoa from the heat and set aside for 5 minutes, then fluff it with a fork.

2. Divide the quinoa between 2 bowls and pour ½ cup of the remaining almond milk in each bowl. Add the stevia, if using. Top each dish with half of the sliced pear and 2 tablespoons of almonds.

CALORIES: 247   TOTAL FAT: 12 G   SATURATED FAT: 0 G   SUGAR: 2 G   CARBOHYDRATES: 31 G

Sweetie Pie Smoothie

Treat your palate to the sweet and spicy flavors of apple pie with this morning maintenance smoothie. If you follow the recipe and it comes out too thick, add some unsweetened almond milk to thin it out. Apple pie spice typically consists of cinnamon, nutmeg, and allspice, but you may certainly make your own blend as you like it.

1½ APPLES, HALVED AND SEEDED

¾ CUP PROBIOTIC YOGURT

⅛ TEASPOON ALCOHOL-FREE
     VANILLA EXTRACT

½ TEASPOON APPLE PIE SPICE

¼ TEASPOON POWDERED STEVIA

1 CUP ICE CUBES

1. Combine all the ingredients in a blender and process until smooth.

2. Divide the smoothie among 3 glasses and enjoy.

CALORIES: 86   TOTAL FAT: 0 G   SATURATED FAT: 0 G   SUGAR: 16 G   CARBOHYDRATES: 20 G

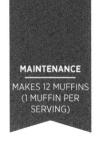

Strawberry Muffins

Great for an on-the-go breakfast or snack, these muffins are a stellar way to celebrate strawberry season in the summer. For a light and airy batch, be sure to not overmix your batter.

1 CUP GROUND FLAXSEED

1 CUP ALMOND FLOUR

1 TABLESPOON GLUTEN-FREE
    BAKING POWDER

1½ TEASPOONS GROUND NUTMEG

1 TEASPOON CINNAMON

¼ TEASPOON SEA SALT

½ CUP (1 STICK) BUTTER, MELTED
    AND COOLED

4 EGGS

6 TEASPOONS POWDERED STEVIA

½ CUP WATER

12 STRAWBERRIES, SLICED

1. Preheat the oven to 350°F.

2. Line a 12-cup muffin pan with paper muffin liners.

3. In a large mixing bowl, whisk together the flaxseed meal, almond flour, baking powder, nutmeg, cinnamon, and salt.

4. In a separate mixing bowl, combine the butter, eggs, stevia, and water.

5. Make a well in the dry ingredients and pour the butter mixture into the center of the well. Stir until the ingredients are just combined.

6. Using an ice cream scoop or a large spoon, distribute the mix evenly into the muffin pan, filling each cup two-thirds full. Place the strawberry slices on top of each cup of batter.

7. Bake the muffins for 20 minutes, or until a toothpick inserted in the center of a muffin comes out clean. Remove the muffins from the muffin pan and allow them to cool completely before serving.

CALORIES: 149   TOTAL FAT: 14 G   SATURATED FAT: 6 G   SUGAR: 1 G   CARBOHYDRATES: 5 G

Blueberry-Lemon Pancakes

Even though these pancakes are a tasty treat, leftovers are always a possibility. Save your extras by placing them in a freezer bag after they have cooled completely. When you're ready to reheat them, place the frozen pancakes in a toaster oven and cook them at about 300°F for one to two minutes, until warm.

2 EGGS, BEATEN

¼ TEASPOON POWDERED STEVIA

2 TABLESPOONS COCONUT OIL, MELTED AND COOLED

¾ CUP UNSWEETENED ALMOND MILK

1½ CUPS ALMOND FLOUR

2 TEASPOONS COCONUT FLOUR

½ TEASPOON GLUTEN-FREE BAKING SODA

1 TEASPOON GLUTEN-FREE BAKING POWDER

¼ TEASPOON SEA SALT

ZEST OF 2 LEMONS

NONSTICK COOKING SPRAY

1 CUP BLUEBERRIES

1. Heat a griddle or a cast-iron skillet over medium heat.

2. Using a blender or food processor, process the eggs, stevia, coconut oil, almond milk, almond flour, coconut flour, baking soda, baking powder, salt, and lemon zest.

3. Spray the skillet with cooking spray and pour ¼ cup of pancake batter at a time into rounds. Top each round with a handful of blueberries. Cook the pancakes until bubbles begin to form on the surface of the pancakes, 1 to 1½ minutes. Using a spatula, flip each pancake over and cook the other side for about 1 minute.

4. Remove the pancakes from the skillet and cover them with a clean towel to keep them warm.

5. Repeat the cooking process until all the pancake batter is used. Serve the pancakes warm, 2 pancakes per serving.

CALORIES: 154   TOTAL FAT: 12 G   SATURATED FAT: 6 G   SUGAR: 4 G   CARBOHYDRATES: 9 G

Coconut Millet with Cacao and Raspberries

Have you surpassed your weekly quinoa quota? No worries—there are plenty of gluten-free grains out there. High in fiber and protein, millet can help you shake up your menu a bit. The nutty grain pairs well with cholesterol-free sunflower seed butter in this comforting breakfast bowl. Cacao nibs are cacao beans that have been roasted, hulled, and prepped to be made into chocolate. They taste a bit like roasted coffee beans and can be found in health food and upscale grocery stores.

6 CUPS WATER

¼ TEASPOON SEA SALT

1 CUP UNCOOKED MILLET

½ CUP UNSWEETENED ALMOND MILK

½ CUP RASPBERRIES

¼ CUP SHREDDED UNSWEETENED COCONUT

3 TEASPOONS CACAO NIBS

4 TABLESPOONS SUNFLOWER SEED BUTTER

1. In a large pot, bring the water and salt to a boil. Pour in the millet and return it to a boil. Reduce the heat, cover, and simmer for 25 to 30 minutes. Remove the pot from the heat and let the millet cool for 5 minutes. Fluff with a fork.

2. Divide the cooked millet among 4 bowls. While it's still warm, top each bowl with almond milk, raspberries, coconut, cacao nibs, and 1 tablespoon of sunflower seed butter.

CALORIES: 340   TOTAL FAT: 13 G   SATURATED FAT: 2 G   SUGAR: 2 G   CARBOHYDRATES: 49 G

Coconut Custard with Pineapple

MAINTENANCE
SERVES 4

You might feel a craving for something sweet and creamy when following the candida diet, so this fruit-topped custard could be the perfect breakfast indulgence. This recipe is simple to make but should be completed the evening before so that the custard has time to chill and firm up. For an alternate flavor, you can top the custards with fresh berries instead of pineapple.

1½ CUPS UNSWEETENED
COCONUT MILK
½ VANILLA BEAN
½ TEASPOON LIQUID STEVIA OR
1 TEASPOON POWDERED STEVIA

PINCH SEA SALT
5 EGG YOLKS
1 CUP FINELY CHOPPED FRESH
PINEAPPLE

1. Preheat the oven to 350°F.

2. Place the coconut milk in a medium saucepan.

3. Use a sharp paring knife to cut the vanilla bean lengthwise, then use the flat of the knife to scrape the seeds into the coconut milk. Add the vanilla bean pod to the milk with the stevia and salt.

4. Heat the mixture over medium-high heat until the milk is steaming but not boiling. Remove the saucepan from the heat.

5. In a small bowl, whisk the egg yolks. Pour about half of the hot milk mixture into the yolks, whisking to combine.

6. Pour the egg mixture back into the rest of the hot coconut milk and whisk to combine.

7. Pour the hot egg mixture through a fine sieve into a bowl or pitcher.

8. Place 4 (6-ounce) custard cups in a baking dish and fill the dish halfway with water.

continued ▶

9. Pour the custard mixture into the cups and cover the entire dish with foil.

10. Carefully place the dish in the oven and bake the custards for 25 to 30 minutes, until the edges of the custards are firm but the centers still jiggle slightly.

11. Remove the custards from the oven and place the ramekins on a wire rack for about 30 minutes to cool.

12. Place the custards in the fridge until they are completely cool, about 1 hour, then cover them with plastic wrap until ready to serve.

13. Serve the custard topped with the pineapple.

CALORIES: 295   TOTAL FAT: 27 G   SATURATED FAT: 21 G   SUGAR: 7 G   CARBOHYDRATES: 11 G

Very Berry Parfait

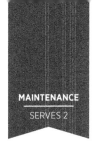

Simple is sometimes best when it comes to a quick breakfast, but that doesn't mean something unhealthy. The yogurt and almonds provide protein, which combines with the carbohydrates in the berries to supply energy all day long. You can put these parfaits together the night before to save time.

16 OUNCES FAT-FREE PLAIN YOGURT

2 CUPS FRESH MIXED BERRIES,
    INCLUDING STRAWBERRIES,
    BLUEBERRIES, AND RASPBERRIES

2 TABLESPOONS CHOPPED
    ROASTED ALMONDS

1. Spoon about 2 tablespoons of yogurt into 2 large parfait or drinking glasses.

2. Top the yogurt with 2 tablespoons of fresh berries.

3. Repeat this layering until all the yogurt and berries have been used.

4. Top each parfait with 1 tablespoon of chopped almonds before serving.

CALORIES: 222   TOTAL FAT: 4 G   SATURATED FAT: 0 G   SUGAR: 26 G   CARBOHYDRATES: 37 G

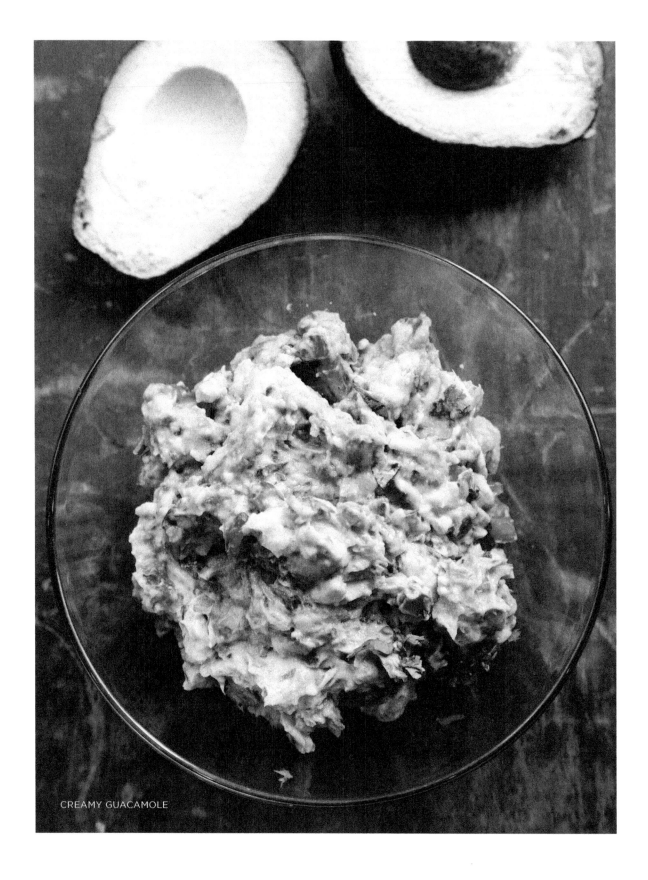

CREAMY GUACAMOLE

6

Snacks

CLEANSE

PUFFED QUINOA TREATS

QUINOA-SESAME BUCKWHEAT CRACKERS

SPICY KALE CHIPS

CAYENNE-SPICED WALNUTS

TRAIL MIX

OVEN-ROASTED ONION-GARLIC DIP

CREAMY GUACAMOLE

GINGERY BRUSSELS SPROUTS

GARLICKY MIXED BITTER GREENS

ROASTED RADICCHIO WITH THYME

CURRIED DEVILED EGGS

SPICY BAKED CHICKEN WINGS

MAINTENANCE

BERRY SKEWERS WITH CHIA-YOGURT DIP

BERRY SAVORY ANTS ON A LOG

MIXED NUT BARS

ROASTED GINGER-CUMIN CHICKPEAS

ROASTED BEET AND GARLIC "HUMMUS"

ROASTED EGGPLANT TAPENADE

SAVORY AND SWEET POTATO CHIPS

COCONUT-LIME SWEET POTATOES

MASHED PARSNIPS AND APPLES

CHICKEN MEATBALLS

Puffed Quinoa Treats

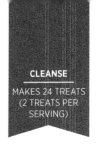
This is a rich treat that will remind you of Rice Krispies squares without all the sugary marshmallow. You can add any nut for the crunch and experiment with unsweetened carob chips, as well, to create delectable variations. If you cannot find puffed quinoa, then puffed brown rice works well too.

1 CUP NO-SUGAR-ADDED
ALMOND BUTTER

2½ CUPS PUFFED QUINOA
2 TABLESPOONS CHOPPED ALMONDS

1. Heat the almond butter in a small saucepan over low heat until it is just melted, about 3 minutes, then remove the pan from the heat.

2. In a medium bowl, combine the melted almond butter, puffed quinoa, and chopped almonds until they are well mixed.

3. Place the bowl in the fridge for about 20 minutes or until the mixture is firm enough to roll into balls.

4. Roll the mixture into 24 balls each about 1½ inches in diameter.

5. Store the treats in the fridge in a sealed container for up to 1 week.

CALORIES: 138   TOTAL FAT: 7 G   SATURATED FAT: 1 G   SUGAR: 1 G   CARBOHYDRATES: 16 G

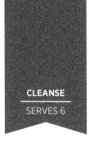

Quinoa-Sesame Buckwheat Crackers

Yes, raw vegetables are crunchy, but there are times when you've simply got to have the crispy crunch of a cracker.

¼ CUP UNCOOKED QUINOA

3¾ CUPS WATER, PLUS 2 TABLESPOONS

½ CUP BUCKWHEAT FLOUR, PLUS MORE FOR DUSTING

½ TEASPOON SEA SALT, PLUS MORE FOR SEASONING

3 TABLESPOONS SESAME SEEDS

2 TABLESPOONS OLIVE OIL, PLUS MORE FOR DRIZZLING

1. Soak the quinoa for 6 to 8 hours in 3 cups of water. Drain and rinse well.

2. Using a small saucepan, bring ¾ cup of water and the quinoa to a boil. Cover and reduce the heat to a simmer. Cook for 10 to 15 minutes, or until the quinoa is tender and the water is absorbed. Set it aside to cool slightly.

3. Preheat the oven to 400°F.

4. Line a baking sheet with parchment paper.

5. Using a food processor, pulse the quinoa a few times. Add in the buckwheat flour and salt, and process until coarse. Add 2 tablespoons of sesame seeds and pulse a few times.

6. With the processor running, slowly add the olive oil and 2 tablespoons of water. Process until a ball forms; the dough should be soft.

7. Flatten and spread the dough on a large rolling surface, creating a 6-inch round. Sprinkle it generously with buckwheat flour. Roll it out with a rolling pin until it is ⅛-inch thick.

8. Using a pastry brush, coat the dough with a drizzle of olive oil. Sprinkle it with salt and the remaining 1 tablespoon of sesame seeds, lightly pressing them in.

9. Bake the cracker for 40 minutes, until it has browned. Remove the cracker from the heat when it is crispy. Allow it to cool before breaking it into 6 pieces.

CALORIES: 137   TOTAL FAT: 8 G   SATURATED FAT: 1 G   SUGAR: 1 G   CARBOHYDRATES: 15 G

Spicy Kale Chips

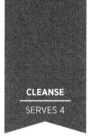

Kale chips can be found in most grocery stores, but it is healthier to put them together yourself. The trick to crispy kale chips is to make sure you dry the kale off very well before tossing it with the other ingredients. You can use any combination of seasonings for kale chips, so experiment to see what works well with your palate.

1 BUNCH KALE, DRIED AND CHOPPED INTO 1-INCH PIECES

3 TEASPOONS OLIVE OIL

½ TEASPOON GARLIC POWDER

¼ TEASPOON SEA SALT

PINCH SMOKED PAPRIKA

1. Preheat the oven to 350°F.

2. Line a baking sheet with parchment paper.

3. In a large bowl, toss together the kale, olive oil, garlic powder, sea salt, and paprika until the kale is well coated.

4. Transfer the kale to the prepared baking sheet and bake it until it is crispy, 10 to 15 minutes.

5. Remove the kale chips from the oven and allow them to cool completely.

6. Kale chips are best fresh, but they can be stored in a sealed container at room temperature for up to 3 days.

CALORIES: 73   TOTAL FAT: 4 G   SATURATED FAT: 1 G   SUGAR: 0 G   CARBOHYDRATES: 9 G

Cayenne-Spiced Walnuts

If there was ever a time to experiment with spice, it's now, when your diet might get a little bland or boring. By getting creative in the kitchen and jazzing up traditional snacks, you can delight your palate while still being candida-free. A handful of these spicy walnuts—which can be stored in an airtight container for a few days—will not only satisfy an afternoon carb craving, but it will also help you feel full longer thanks to a healthy dose of good fat and fiber.

NONSTICK COOKING SPRAY

1 EGG WHITE

1 TEASPOON CAYENNE PEPPER

1 TEASPOON PAPRIKA

1 TEASPOON DRIED OREGANO

1 TEASPOON DRIED THYME

½ TEASPOON SEA SALT

12 OUNCES WALNUTS

1. Preheat the oven to 350°F.

2. Coat a baking sheet with cooking spray.

3. In a large mixing bowl, whisk together the egg white, cayenne pepper, paprika, oregano, thyme, and salt. Stir in the walnuts until well combined.

4. Spread the walnuts in a single layer on the baking sheet and bake them for 15 to 18 minutes, until crispy.

CALORIES: 186   TOTAL FAT: 18 G   SATURATED FAT: 2 G   SUGAR: 1 G   CARBOHYDRATES: 4 G

Trail Mix

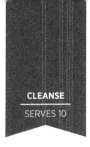
The pumpkin seeds in this energy-packed trail mix are effective candida fighters because they are a natural antifungal due to their high omega-3 fatty acid content. This important nutrient is also great for the skin, and it can fight depression, which can be a problem when dealing with candida.

1 CUP ROASTED SUNFLOWER SEEDS

½ CUP PUMPKIN SEEDS

½ CUP CHOPPED PECANS

½ CUP HAZELNUTS

½ CUP SLIVERED ALMONDS

½ CUP SHREDDED UNSWEETENED
    COCONUT

1. In a large bowl, mix together the sunflower seeds, pumpkin seeds, pecans, hazelnuts, almonds, and coconut until they are well combined.

2. Store the trail mix in a sealed plastic bag at room temperature for up to 1 week or in the freezer for up to 1 month.

CALORIES: 144   TOTAL FAT: 13 G   SATURATED FAT: 3 G   SUGAR: 1 G   CARBOHYDRATES: 5 G

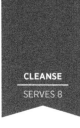

Oven-Roasted Onion-Garlic Dip

Powdered onion dips are a thing of the past! Roasting the onions and garlic extracts a sweet, caramelized flavor that is truly a simple pleasure. Serve this savory delight with Quinoa-Sesame Buckwheat Crackers (page 98) or carrot and celery sticks.

2 SWEET ONIONS, QUARTERED

1 TABLESPOON OLIVE OIL

1 TEASPOON SEA SALT

1 WHOLE HEAD GARLIC

⅓ CUP PLAIN GREEK YOGURT

¼ CUP CHOPPED FRESH PARSLEY

1 TABLESPOON FRESHLY SQUEEZED
LEMON JUICE

1. Preheat the oven to 425°F.

2. Put the onions in a medium mixing bowl, drizzle them with the olive oil, and sprinkle them with ½ teaspoon of salt. Toss to coat.

3. Remove the papery white outer layer from the garlic head, without separating the cloves. Wrap the head in foil.

4. Put the onions and foil-wrapped garlic on a baking sheet. Roast them for 1 hour, then allow them to cool for 10 minutes.

5. Chop the onions. Separate the garlic cloves, and squeeze each clove to extract the pulp. Discard the skins.

6. In a large mixing bowl, combine the onions, garlic, remaining ½ teaspoon of salt, yogurt, parsley, and lemon juice. Cover the dip and chill it for at least 1 hour before serving.

CALORIES: 66   TOTAL FAT: 3 G   SATURATED FAT: 1 G   SUGAR: 2 G   CARBOHYDRATES: 10 G

Creamy Guacamole

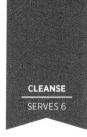

Avocados are an extremely healthy ingredient in your candida diet plan, so it is important to know how to pick and store them. Look for avocados that have no sunken or dark spots on them. The best way to buy avocados is slightly unripe; they ripen easily at home and you can make sure they don't get bruised. After the fruit are ripe, you can store them in the fridge.

2 AVOCADOS, PEELED AND PITTED

¼ RED ONION, PEELED AND
    FINELY DICED

1 TEASPOON MINCED GARLIC

JUICE OF 1 LIME

1 TOMATO, DICED

2 TABLESPOONS CHOPPED
    FRESH CILANTRO

SEA SALT

1. In a medium bowl, add the avocados, onion, garlic, and lime juice and mash the mixture with a fork until it is well mixed but still chunky.

2. Add the tomato and cilantro and stir to combine.

3. Season the mixture with salt.

4. Transfer the guacamole to a sealed container and chill it in the fridge for up to 5 days. Serve it with sliced vegetables or rice cakes.

CALORIES: 141   TOTAL FAT: 13 G   SATURATED FAT: 3 G   SUGAR: 1 G   CARBOHYDRATES: 7 G

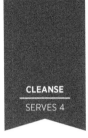

Gingery Brussels Sprouts

Steaming the Brussels sprouts helps boost their cholesterol-lowering powers. Brussels sprouts are also high in vitamins A, C, and K.

1 TABLESPOON COCONUT OIL

1 ONION, THINLY SLICED

2 GARLIC CLOVES, MINCED

1 (1-INCH) PIECE FRESH GINGER, JULIENNED

2 POUNDS BRUSSELS SPROUTS, SHREDDED

3 TABLESPOONS WATER

SEA SALT

FRESHLY GROUND BLACK PEPPER

1. Heat a large sauté pan over medium-high heat. Coat the pan with the coconut oil, then add the onion, garlic, and ginger and sauté for 2 to 3 minutes.

2. Add the Brussels sprouts and 2 tablespoons of water. Cover and cook for 10 to 15 minutes, or until the sprouts are tender.

3. Add the remaining 1 tablespoon of water and season the sprouts with salt and pepper. Serve warm.

CALORIES: 100   TOTAL FAT: 4 G   SATURATED FAT: 3 G   SUGAR: 3 G   CARBOHYDRATES: 15 G

Garlicky Mixed Bitter Greens

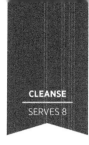

Bitter foods help reduce your craving for sugar, and this recipe has loads of them. The kale, broccoli rabe, and collard greens are all packed with nutrients, and the bitterness mellows a bit with cooking.

1 CUP LOW-SODIUM GLUTEN-FREE
    CHICKEN BROTH
¾ CUP SLICED LEEKS, WHITE
    PARTS ONLY
½ CUP CHOPPED SCALLIONS
1 TABLESPOON MINCED GARLIC
3 CUPS CHOPPED KALE

1 CUP CHOPPED BROCCOLI RABE
3 CUPS CHOPPED COLLARD GREENS
1 TABLESPOON OLIVE OIL
SEA SALT
¼ TEASPOON FRESHLY GROUND
    BLACK PEPPER

1. In a large skillet over medium-high heat, heat 1 tablespoon of broth. Add the leeks, scallions, and garlic. Sauté until the leeks are limp, about 4 minutes.

2. Add the kale, broccoli rabe, and collard greens and cook, stirring constantly, until the greens wilt, about 10 minutes. Add the remaining broth and simmer, stirring occasionally, until the greens are tender, about 15 minutes.

3. Drizzle the greens with the olive oil and season them with salt and pepper.

CALORIES: 46   TOTAL FAT: 2 G   SATURATED FAT: 1 G   SUGAR: 1 G   CARBOHYDRATES: 6 G

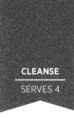
Roasted Radicchio with Thyme

Bitter vegetables like radicchio are great for the cleanse. When you cut the radicchio into wedges, make sure to leave some of the core attached to each section; this will hold the leaves together while the dish is cooking.

2 HEADS OF RADICCHIO (ABOUT 1 POUND TOTAL), HALVED THROUGH THE CORE AND CUT INTO THREE WEDGES PER HALF

3 TABLESPOONS OLIVE OIL

1 TABLESPOON CHOPPED FRESH THYME

SEA SALT

FRESHLY GROUND BLACK PEPPER

1. Preheat the oven to 450°F.

2. Wash the radicchio wedges and shake off some of the water (leave some of the water on the leaves). Drizzle the radicchio wedges with olive oil, sprinkle them with thyme, and season them with salt and pepper. Toss the radicchio wedges gently until they are evenly coated.

3. Place the wedges on a baking sheet with 1 of the cut sides facing up. Roast for 12 minutes or until the wedges are wilted.

4. Turn the wedges over so the other cut side is facing up and roast them for 8 minutes more, or until tender.

CALORIES: 104   TOTAL FAT: 11 G   SATURATED FAT: 2 G   SUGAR: 1 G   CARBOHYDRATES: 3 G

Curried Deviled Eggs

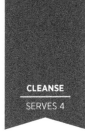

These traditional snacks are not technically deviled because you will be using yogurt instead of mayonnaise for the filling, but the end result is close enough to keep the name. The yogurt is tarter than mayonnaise, but the addition of curry makes that difference unnoticeable. You can adjust the heat in the eggs by using either hot or mild curry powder.

6 BOILED EGGS, COOLED AND PEELED
¼ CUP PLAIN GREEK YOGURT
1 TABLESPOON FRESHLY SQUEEZED
    LEMON JUICE
½ TEASPOON CURRY POWDER

PINCH DRY MUSTARD
SEA SALT
FRESHLY GROUND BLACK PEPPER
2 TABLESPOONS CHOPPED
    FRESH CHIVES

1. Cut the eggs in half lengthwise and carefully scoop the cooked yolks out into a small bowl.

2. Place the empty white halves on a serving plate and set aside.

3. Use a fork to mash the yolks.

4. Add the yogurt, lemon juice, curry, and mustard to the mashed yolks, stirring until the mixture is well blended and fluffy.

5. Season the mixture with salt and pepper.

6. Scoop the mixture evenly back into the egg whites and top the deviled eggs with the chives, dividing evenly.

7. Chill the eggs in the fridge covered with plastic wrap for up to 2 days.

CALORIES: 129   TOTAL FAT: 8 G   SATURATED FAT: 2 G   SUGAR: 3 G   CARBOHYDRATES: 5 G

Spicy Baked Chicken Wings

Battling a craving for something spicy? Bake up some chicken wings to satisfy your savory need in a healthy way. If you prefer mild wings, omit the jalapeño pepper.

¼ CUP COCONUT OIL

½ TEASPOON FINELY MINCED GARLIC

2 TABLESPOONS FINELY
   MINCED ONION

¼ TEASPOON MINCED FRESH
   CILANTRO

1 TABLESPOON FINELY MINCED
   JALAPEÑO PEPPER

¼ TEASPOON SEA SALT

¼ CUP NO-SALT, NO-SUGAR-ADDED
   TOMATO PASTE

PINCH STEVIA

⅛ CUP FRESHLY SQUEEZED
   LEMON JUICE

2 POUNDS CHICKEN WINGS

1. Preheat the oven to 375°F.

2. In a large saucepan over medium heat, melt the coconut oil. Stir in the garlic, onion, cilantro, and jalapeño pepper. Sauté the mixture until the onions and jalapeño pepper are tender, about 6 minutes.

3. In a separate saucepan, combine the salt, tomato paste, stevia, and lemon juice. Simmer the mixture for 5 minutes.

4. Add the tomato paste mixture to the coconut oil mixture and bring it to a boil, stirring constantly, until it thickens.

5. Remove the saucepan from the heat and allow it to cool.

6. In a large mixing bowl, toss the sauce with the chicken wings until well combined. Spread the wings on a large baking sheet. Roast the wings for 30 minutes, shaking the pan halfway through cooking. If you have extra sauce, use it to baste the wings when they are almost done.

CALORIES: 227   TOTAL FAT: 12 G   SATURATED FAT: 7 G   SUGAR: 1 G   CARBOHYDRATES: 2 G

Berry Skewers with Chia-Yogurt Dip

Although ripe berries taste sweet, they are still considered low in sugar and may help you overcome a craving for dessert. Not only will this snack give you a fruity fix, but it will also give you an additional boost of omega-3 fatty acids, protein, calcium, and fiber, thanks to the chia seeds in the dip.

8 OUNCES STRAWBERRIES, TOPS TRIMMED

6 OUNCES RASPBERRIES

6 OUNCES BLUEBERRIES

1 CUP PLAIN GREEK YOGURT

½ TEASPOON ALCOHOL-FREE VANILLA EXTRACT

3 TEASPOONS CHIA SEEDS

1. Using a food processor, purée the strawberries, 3 ounces of raspberries, and 3 ounces of blueberries.

2. In a large mixing bowl, combine the berry purée, yogurt, vanilla, and 2 teaspoons of chia seeds. Chill the dip for 15 minutes, or until it has thickened.

3. Arrange the remaining berries on skewers. Top off the yogurt dip with the remaining 1 teaspoon of chia seeds before serving. Serve the skewers alongside the dip.

CALORIES: 39   TOTAL FAT: 1 G   SATURATED FAT: 0 G   SUGAR: 4 G   CARBOHYDRATES: 6 G

Berry Savory Ants on a Log

When it comes to healthy snacks, your parents may have been onto something. This updated version of an old standby is better than ever, thanks to the fresh fruit and heart-healthy almond butter.

½ CUP NO-SUGAR-ADDED
    ALMOND BUTTER
4 CELERY STALKS

¼ CUP BLUEBERRIES
2 TABLESPOONS SUNFLOWER SEEDS

1. Spread the almond butter inside the celery stalks.

2. Top each celery stalk with blueberries and sunflower seeds. Cut each stalk into quarters.

CALORIES: 107   TOTAL FAT: 9 G   SATURATED FAT: 1 G   SUGAR: 1 G   CARBOHYDRATES: 4 G

Mixed Nut Bars

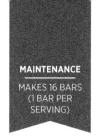

Commercially prepared granola bars are packed with sugar and other ingredients that are not allowed on a candida diet, like dried fruit and chocolate. Candida-friendly nut bars are filling and can be a quick energy snack after a workout or when you hit a midafternoon energy slump.

1 CUP NO-SUGAR-ADDED
    ALMOND BUTTER
½ CUP COCONUT OIL
1 CUP OAT BRAN
1 CUP SESAME SEEDS

1 CUP SHREDDED UNSWEETENED
    COCONUT
½ CUP CHOPPED HAZELNUTS
½ CUP CHOPPED PECANS
½ CUP SUNFLOWER SEEDS
1 TEASPOON GROUND CINNAMON

1. Line a 9-by-13-inch glass pan with parchment paper and set aside.

2. Place the almond butter and coconut oil in a small saucepan over medium heat and stir until they melt, about 4 minutes. Remove the saucepan from the heat.

3. In a large bowl, stir together the oat bran, sesame seeds, shredded coconut, hazelnuts, pecans, sunflower seeds, and cinnamon.

4. Pour the melted almond butter into the nut mixture and stir until it is well mixed.

5. Transfer the bar batter to the prepared pan and spread it out evenly. Press the nut mixture down firmly and place the pan in the fridge until it is cool and set, about 2 hours.

6. Turn the hardened mixture out onto a cutting board and cut it into 16 bars.

7. Store the bars in a sealed container in the fridge for up to 1 week or in the freezer for up to 2 months.

CALORIES: 289   TOTAL FAT: 27 G   SATURATED FAT: 10 G   SUGAR: 1 G   CARBOHYDRATES: 11 G

Roasted Ginger-Cumin Chickpeas

If you're missing the crunch of crackers and potato chips, crispy chickpeas are the way to go. Low in fat and high in fiber, they are a savory snack that actually makes you feel full longer. Go ahead and make a double batch—they can be stored in an airtight container for up to two weeks.

1 (15-OUNCE) CAN SODIUM-FREE CHICKPEAS, DRAINED AND RINSED

1 TABLESPOON OLIVE OIL

¼ TEASPOON GROUND CUMIN

¼ TEASPOON GROUND CORIANDER

¼ TEASPOON GROUND GINGER

¼ TEASPOON PAPRIKA

½ TEASPOON SEA SALT

1. Preheat the oven to 425°F.

2. In a medium mixing bowl, toss the chickpeas with the olive oil, cumin, coriander, ginger, paprika, and salt until well combined.

3. Spread the chickpeas evenly on a baking sheet and roast them for about 30 minutes, shaking the pan occasionally.

4. Remove the baking sheet from the oven when the chickpeas are golden and crunchy. Let them cool before serving.

CALORIES: 156   TOTAL FAT: 5 G   SATURATED FAT: 1 G   SUGAR: 0 G   CARBOHYDRATES: 24 G

Roasted Beet and Garlic "Hummus"

Say good-bye to the afternoon slump with this protein-rich snack. Between the beets and the white beans, this variation on traditional hummus will provide your body with plenty of energy as well as a blast of vitamins and nutrients. Serve the beautifully bright dish with a side of fennel or celery for dipping.

1 GARLIC CLOVE, CHOPPED

⅓ CUP CHOPPED ROASTED BEETS

1 CUP COOKED WHITE BEANS

2 TABLESPOONS FRESHLY SQUEEZED
    LEMON JUICE

2 TABLESPOONS OLIVE OIL

SEA SALT

FRESHLY GROUND BLACK PEPPER

1. In a food processor, purée the garlic, beets, beans, lemon juice, and oil.

2. Transfer the mixture to a bowl. Season the hummus with salt and pepper.

CALORIES: 236   TOTAL FAT: 8 G   SATURATED FAT: 1 G   SUGAR: 1 G   CARBOHYDRATES: 32 G

Roasted Eggplant Tapenade

Many people don't like eggplant because it can be bitter and has an unusual spongy texture. This tapenade addresses both those potential issues and creates a rich dish that can be used as a dip, a spread on rice cakes, or tossed with rice noodles as a sauce. You can easily double the recipe and freeze the extra for later.

2 EGGPLANTS, CUT INTO
    ½-INCH SLICES
½ TEASPOON SEA SALT
1 RED ONION, PEELED AND CHOPPED
3 GARLIC CLOVES, CRUSHED
3 PLUM TOMATOES, CORED AND
    CUT IN HALF
2 TABLESPOONS OLIVE OIL

JUICE OF ½ LEMON
1 TEASPOON CHOPPED
    FRESH OREGANO
1 TEASPOON CHOPPED FRESH BASIL
¼ CUP CHOPPED BLACK OLIVES
1 TABLESPOON CHOPPED FRESH
    PARSLEY, FOR GARNISH

1. Preheat the oven to 350°F.

2. Spread the eggplant slices on a baking sheet and sprinkle them with salt to draw out the bitterness. Let the eggplant sit for 30 minutes, then blot it with a paper towel.

3. Place the onion, garlic, and tomatoes on the baking sheet with the eggplant and drizzle them with the olive oil and lemon juice.

4. Bake the mixture in the oven until the vegetables are tender, about 50 minutes.

5. Let the vegetables cool on the baking sheet, then transfer them to a food processor.

6. Pulse until the vegetables are coarsely diced, then transfer the mixture to a medium bowl.

7. Stir in the herbs and olives and garnish with the parsley.

8. Store the tapenade in the fridge for up to 5 days.

CALORIES: 126   TOTAL FAT: 7 G   SATURATED FAT: 1 G   SUGAR: 7 G   CARBOHYDRATES: 15 G

Savory and Sweet Potato Chips

MAINTENANCE
SERVES 4

These tasty sweet potato bites will not only give you something crunchy to snack on but will also deliver a punch of potassium, calcium, and vitamins A and C. A mandoline may be the best and quickest way to slice up the sweet potatoes, but you may also prepare them for baking with a sharp knife and a little patience. Feel free to add cayenne pepper to the spice mix to amp up the flavor, or serve the chips with a side of lemon wedges.

1 SWEET POTATO, PEELED AND VERY
    THINLY SLICED

1 TABLESPOON OLIVE OIL

GROUND CUMIN

PAPRIKA

SEA SALT

1. Preheat the oven to 400°F.

2. In a large mixing bowl, coat the sweet potato slices with the oil and season them with the cumin, paprika, and salt.

3. Using 2 baking sheets, arrange the sweet potato slices in a single layer and bake them for 20 to 25 minutes, stirring them halfway through the cooking time, and switching the position of the baking sheets in the oven at the same time.

4. Remove the baking sheets from the oven when the chips are crisp and golden.

CALORIES: 56   TOTAL FAT: 4 G   SATURATED FAT: 1 G   SUGAR: 2 G   CARBOHYDRATES: 6 G

Coconut-Lime Sweet Potatoes

Sweet potatoes are more nutritious than their paler cousins. They are full of calcium, potassium, and vitamins. Roasting them heightens their natural sugars and make them taste almost like a dessert.

2 TABLESPOONS COCONUT OIL

2 POUNDS SWEET POTATOES, PEELED AND CUT INTO 1-INCH CHUNKS

½ TEASPOON SEA SALT

¼ TEASPOON FRESHLY GROUND BLACK PEPPER

1 TEASPOON GRATED LIME ZEST

1. Preheat the oven to 400°F.

2. In a small saucepan over medium heat, melt the coconut oil. Toss the potatoes with the oil, salt, and pepper.

3. Spread the potatoes in a single layer on a large baking sheet. Roast the potatoes, stirring occasionally, until tender, about 40 minutes.

4. Toss the potatoes with the lime zest and serve.

CALORIES: 162   TOTAL FAT: 8 G   SATURATED FAT: 6 G   SUGAR: 0 G   CARBOHYDRATES: 24 G

Mashed Parsnips and Apples

Puréed parsnips are a worthy substitute for a cozy side of creamy mashed potatoes. When shopping for apples for this recipe, seek out a tart variety, like Honeycrisp, which hold up the best. If you need to alter the consistency of the mash, add water or chicken broth until it's as you like it.

5 PARSNIPS, PEELED

3 APPLES, PEELED, CORED, AND CUT
   INTO 1-INCH PIECES

4 TABLESPOONS BUTTER, AT ROOM
   TEMPERATURE

SEA SALT

FRESHLY GROUND BLACK PEPPER

GROUND NUTMEG

1. Preheat the oven to 350°F.

2. Cut each parsnip in half. Chop the thin ends into 1-inch pieces. Quarter the larger halves, remove and discard the tough core, and then chop the remaining halves into 1-inch pieces.

3. Toss the apples, parsnips, and butter in a large bowl, thoroughly coating the apples and parsnips. Transfer everything to a 9-by-13-inch baking dish.

4. Bake the apples and parsnips for 45 minutes, stirring after 30 minutes.

5. Turn up heat to 425°F and bake the apples and parsnips for an additional 20 minutes, until all the liquid has evaporated. When the apples and parsnips have started to brown and caramelize, remove them from the oven.

6. Using a food processor or a blender, process the parsnips and apples until smooth. Season the mixture with salt and pepper and sprinkle it with nutmeg. Serve warm or at room temperature.

CALORIES: 198 TOTAL FAT: 8 G SATURATED FAT: 5 G SUGAR: 15 G CARBOHYDRATES: 33 G

Chicken Meatballs

Savory herbed meatballs are the perfect snack to bring to a potluck dinner or to serve during a backyard barbeque. You can also add them to a homemade tomato sauce served over rice noodles on pasta night. Take care to watch the meatballs carefully when they are in the oven, because the chicken is very lean and they can dry out if cooked too long.

1 TEASPOON OLIVE OIL

1 SWEET ONION, PEELED AND
    FINELY DICED

2 TEASPOONS MINCED GARLIC

1 POUND GROUND LEAN
    CHICKEN BREAST

1 EGG YOLK

2 TABLESPOONS CHOPPED
    FRESH PARSLEY

1 TEASPOON CHOPPED FRESH THYME

¼ TEASPOON FRESHLY GROUND
    BLACK PEPPER

1. Preheat the oven to 400°F.

2. Line a baking sheet with parchment paper. Set aside.

3. In a small skillet over medium heat, combine the olive oil, onion, and garlic, and sauté them until softened, about 3 minutes. Transfer the onion and garlic to a large bowl.

4. Add the chicken breast, egg yolk, parsley, thyme, and pepper to the bowl and mix until everything is well combined.

5. Form the mixture into meatballs, each about 1½ inches in diameter, and place them on the baking sheet.

6. Bake the meatballs until they are completely cooked through, about 15 minutes. Serve immediately.

CALORIES: 166   TOTAL FAT: 5 G   SATURATED FAT: 1 G   SUGAR: 1 G   CARBOHYDRATES: 3 G

NOTES

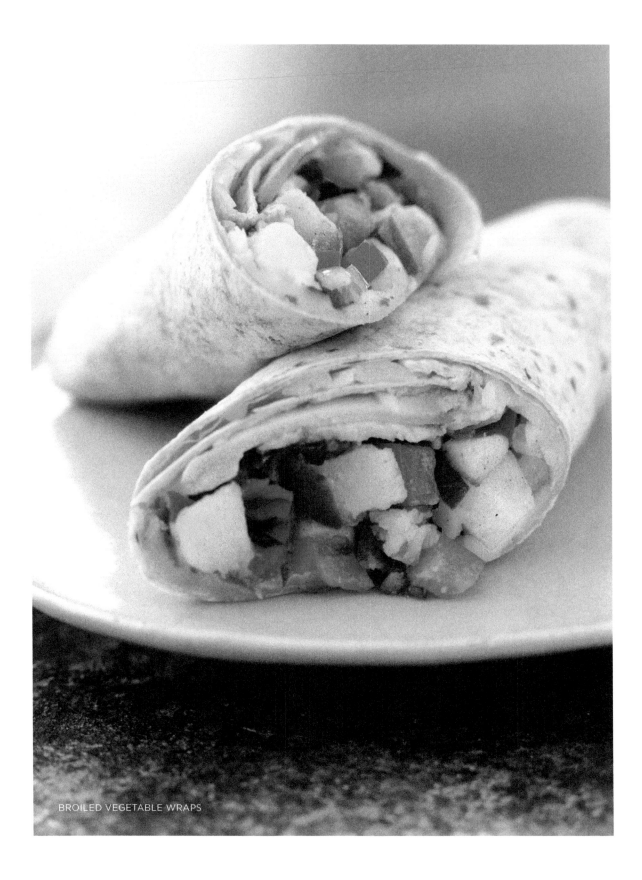

BROILED VEGETABLE WRAPS

7

Soups and Sandwiches

CLEANSE

SPINACH-CELERIAC SOUP

CREAM OF ROASTED CAULIFLOWER SOUP

TOMATO FLORENTINE SOUP

CLASSIC EGG DROP SOUP

ALMOND BUTTER BREAD

OPEN-FACED CUCUMBER SANDWICHES

PRIMAVERA EGG SANDWICHES

LEMON-SALMON SANDWICHES

MAINTENANCE

MEXICAN-SPICED TOMATO AND WHITE BEAN SOUP

CHICKEN AND SWEET POTATO SOUP WITH COLLARD GREENS

BEEF AND VEGETABLE STEW

BROILED VEGETABLE WRAPS

GROUND LAMB AND LENTIL LETTUCE WRAPS

PESTO CHICKEN LETTUCE ROLLS

GREEK-STYLE STEAK SANDWICHES

Spinach-Celeriac Soup

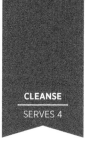

While it may seem hard to believe, there is a candida-, cholesterol-, and dairy-free way of making your soups creamy: Just add puréed celeriac. This miracle root is fat-free and low-calorie while being a good source of vitamin C, iron, and calcium.

2 TABLESPOONS OLIVE OIL
1 GARLIC CLOVE, CRUSHED AND
    FINELY CHOPPED
1 SHALLOT, FINELY CHOPPED
3 CELERY STALKS, CHOPPED
1 CELERIAC BULB, PEELED AND DICED
½ TEASPOON DRIED THYME

4 CUPS LOW-SODIUM GLUTEN-FREE
    CHICKEN BROTH
2 CUPS PACKED BABY SPINACH
2 TEASPOONS FRESHLY SQUEEZED
    LEMON JUICE
½ TEASPOON SEA SALT
FRESHLY GROUND BLACK PEPPER
CHOPPED CHIVES (OPTIONAL)

1. Heat the olive oil in a Dutch oven or a large stockpot, then sauté the garlic and shallot for 2 minutes.

2. Stir in the celery, celeriac, and thyme, and sauté them for 2 minutes.

3. Pour in the broth and bring it to a boil. Reduce the heat and simmer, covered, for 10 minutes, until the vegetables are tender.

4. Stir in the spinach and cook for 2 minutes, or until the spinach has softened.

5. Transfer the mixture to a blender (or use an immersion blender) and purée it until smooth.

6. Add the lemon juice and season with salt and pepper. Garnish with the chives (if using). The soup may be served hot or chilled.

CALORIES: 140   TOTAL FAT: 9 G   SATURATED FAT: 2 G   SUGAR: 2 G   CARBOHYDRATES: 10 G

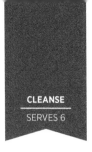

Cream of Roasted Cauliflower Soup

The list of nutrients packed into cauliflower is long and impressive, making it a worthy addition to your diet. When puréed, the white cruciferous florets become airy and almost creamy, creating a dairy-free indulgence. Of course, the unsweetened coconut milk adds to the creamy consistency.

1 HEAD (ABOUT 2½ POUNDS) CAULIFLOWER

14 GARLIC CLOVES, WHOLE AND PEELED

4 TABLESPOONS OLIVE OIL

¾ TEASPOON SEA SALT

¼ TEASPOON FRESHLY GROUND BLACK PEPPER

1 CUP THINLY SLICED LEEK, WHITE AND LIGHT-GREEN PARTS

½ CUP CHOPPED CARROT

½ CUP CHOPPED CELERY

1 TEASPOON DRIED THYME

3 CUPS LOW-SODIUM GLUTEN-FREE CHICKEN OR VEGETABLE BROTH

1 (15-OUNCE) CAN UNSWEETENED COCONUT MILK

1. Preheat the oven to 400°F.

2. Cut the cauliflower head into small florets, discarding the outer green leaves and core. In a large mixing bowl, toss the cauliflower florets with the garlic cloves, 3 tablespoons of olive oil, salt, and pepper. Transfer the mixture to a large baking dish.

3. Roast the cauliflower mixture for about 30 minutes, or until the florets are tender and the edges start to brown, stirring halfway through the cooking time.

4. While the cauliflower cooks, add the remaining 1 tablespoon of olive oil to a large stockpot. Brown the leek, carrot, celery, and thyme over medium-high heat, 7 to 8 minutes.

5. Cover the pot and cook the vegetables for 10 minutes, or until the vegetables are tender.

6. Add the roasted cauliflower to the stockpot, then pour in the broth. Bring the soup to almost a boil, then turn the heat down and simmer for 10 minutes.

7. Transfer the soup to a blender (or use an immersion blender) and purée it until smooth.

8. Add in the coconut milk and mix well. Season with additional salt and pepper if desired.

CALORIES: 299   TOTAL FAT: 27 G   SATURATED FAT: 17 G   SUGAR: 5 G   CARBOHYDRATES: 13 G

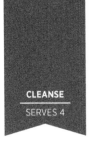
Tomato Florentine Soup

Don't let a candida-free diet keep you from enjoying some of your favorite comfort foods. Quick and easy, this tomato soup requires little prep time, making it a great midweek meal. If you prefer a creamy soup, process it with an immersion blender—before you stir in the spinach—and mix in a small dollop of plain Greek yogurt.

2 TABLESPOONS OLIVE OIL

1 SHALLOT, FINELY CHOPPED

2 GARLIC CLOVES, CHOPPED

1 (28-OUNCE) CAN DICED TOMATOES
    IN JUICE, DRAINED

1 (28-OUNCE) CAN CRUSHED
    TOMATOES

2 CUPS LOW-SODIUM GLUTEN-FREE
    VEGETABLE STOCK

5 OUNCES BABY SPINACH

SEA SALT

FRESHLY GROUND BLACK PEPPER

1. In a stockpot or a Dutch oven, heat the oil and sauté the shallot and garlic over medium heat for 5 minutes.

2. Stir in the diced and the crushed tomatoes. Pour in the stock and stir until everything is well combined. Bring the soup to a boil, reduce the heat, and simmer for 10 to 15 minutes.

3. Stir in the spinach and cook until it is just wilted, 2 to 3 minutes. Season with salt and pepper.

CALORIES: 217   TOTAL FAT: 8 G   SATURATED FAT: 1 G   SUGAR: 18 G   CARBOHYDRATES: 28 G

Classic Egg Drop Soup

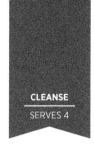

If you don't have time to make your own stock, you may use the store-bought organic kind, but be mindful of the ingredients list. Pass on packaged stock that contains cane sugar or unrecognizable ingredients, and go for a simple list of chicken, water, and vegetables. When preparing this dish, feel free to sneak in some extra greens by stirring in some spinach along with the scallions.

4 CUPS LOW-SODIUM GLUTEN-FREE
   CHICKEN STOCK

2 EGGS, LIGHTLY BEATEN

3 TABLESPOONS CHOPPED SCALLIONS

¼ TEASPOON SEA SALT

1. In a medium saucepan, bring the stock to a boil. Reduce the heat to low.

2. Place a mesh sieve over the pan. Pour the eggs through the sieve and strain them into the soup.

3. Stir in the scallions and salt, and remove the soup from the heat immediately.

CALORIES: 54   TOTAL FAT: 3 G   SATURATED FAT: 1 G   SUGAR: 0 G   CARBOHYDRATES: 2 G

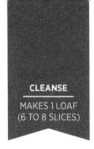
Almond Butter Bread

If you're missing bread, whip up a loaf of this candida-safe option. As a main dish, pair it with Avocado-Basil Chicken Salad (page 148), or fortify a snack by pairing it with Herbed Chicken with White Beans (page 183).

¼ CUP NO-SUGAR-ADDED
    ALMOND BUTTER

4 EGGS

SEA SALT

1 TEASPOON GLUTEN-FREE
    BAKING SODA

NONSTICK COOKING SPRAY

1. Preheat the oven to 325°F.

2. Whisk together the almond butter and eggs until smooth. Add in the salt and baking soda, and mix until well combined.

3. Spray an 8-by-4-inch loaf pan with cooking spray. Pour in the batter. Bake the bread for 30 minutes, until a toothpick inserted in the center comes out clean.

4. Remove the bread from the oven and allow it to cool before slicing it.

(PER LOAF) CALORIES: 649   TOTAL FAT: 53 G   SATURATED FAT: 9 G   SUGAR: 1 G   CARBOHYDRATES: 12 G

Open-Faced Cucumber Sandwiches

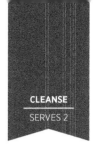

There are many prepared breads you can find in major grocery stores that are appropriate for the candida diet. The bread should be yeast-free and gluten-free. You can also make your own bread for the sandwiches found in this cookbook and your own variations. Good sources for candida-friendly bread recipes are Paleo cookbooks.

4 SLICES YEAST-FREE GLUTEN-
    FREE BREAD

2 TABLESPOONS HOMEMADE BLENDER
    MAYONNAISE (PAGE 30)

1 CUCUMBER, THINLY SLICED

1 AVOCADO, PEELED, PITTED, AND
    THINLY SLICED

4 RADISHES, THINLY SLICED

SEA SALT

FRESHLY GROUND BLACK PEPPER

1 CUP ALFALFA SPROUTS

1. Lay the bread on a clean work surface and spread each slice with mayonnaise.

2. Layer each slice of bread with the cucumber, avocado, and radishes, dividing evenly.

3. Season each open-faced sandwich with salt and pepper.

4. Top each sandwich with ¼ cup of alfalfa sprouts.

5. Serve 2 slices per person.

CALORIES: 397   TOTAL FAT: 27 G   SATURATED FAT: 5 G   SUGAR: 2 G   CARBOHYDRATES: 36 G

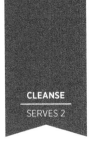
Primavera Egg Sandwiches

The vegetables in this hearty sandwich are tender-crisp, which adds a great deal of texture to the creamy eggs. You can use any candida diet-friendly vegetable for your sandwich, such as leeks, asparagus, and bok choy.

3 TEASPOONS BUTTER

2 GREEN ONIONS, THINLY SLICED

½ CUP CHOPPED BROCCOLI

1 ZUCCHINI, THINLY SLICED

6 EGGS

1 TOMATO, DICED

1 TABLESPOON CHOPPED BASIL

½ TEASPOON CHOPPED THYME

SEA SALT

FRESHLY GROUND BLACK PEPPER

4 SLICES YEAST-FREE GLUTEN-FREE BREAD

1. Place a large skillet over medium-high heat and melt 2 teaspoons of butter.

2. Sauté the green onions, broccoli, and zucchini in the butter until softened, about 3 minutes.

3. In a small bowl, beat the eggs with the tomato and herbs.

4. Pour the egg mixture into the skillet and stir gently with a heat-proof spatula or wooden spoon.

5. As the egg begins to set, lift the edges and push them slightly toward the center, allowing the uncooked egg to flow underneath. Continue this process until the eggs are completely cooked and fluffy, 2 to 3 minutes.

6. Fold the omelet in half, then cut it in half.

7. Season the omelet with salt and pepper.

8. Toast the bread slices and butter them lightly.

9. Place 2 of the bread slices on a clean work surface, then cover each with 1 omelet half. Top each omelet half with another piece of bread. Serve immediately.

CALORIES: 377   TOTAL FAT: 21 G   SATURATED FAT: 8 G   SUGAR: 4 G   CARBOHYDRATES: 26 G

Lemon-Salmon Sandwiches

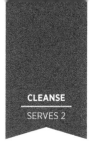

This sandwich filling can also be made with fresh salmon if you have leftovers from other recipes or want to cook some fillets specifically for this recipe. If you are using fresh salmon, choose wild-caught from a reputable source.

1 (5-OUNCE) CAN SALMON, PACKED IN WATER, DRAINED

3 TABLESPOONS HOMEMADE BLENDER MAYONNAISE (PAGE 30)

1 GREEN ONION, FINELY CHOPPED

1 TABLESPOON FRESHLY SQUEEZED LEMON JUICE

1 TEASPOON CHOPPED FRESH DILL

SEA SALT

FRESHLY GROUND BLACK PEPPER

4 SLICES YEAST-FREE GLUTEN-FREE BREAD

1 CUP SHREDDED BOSTON LETTUCE

1. In a medium bowl, combine the salmon, mayonnaise, green onion, lemon juice, and dill until it is well mixed.

2. Season the mixture with salt and pepper.

3. Place 2 of the bread slices on a clean work surface and divide the salmon mixture evenly between them.

4. Top the salmon mixture with shredded lettuce and the other slices of bread. Serve immediately.

CALORIES: 338   TOTAL FAT: 15 G   SATURATED FAT: 2 G   SUGAR: 4 G   CARBOHYDRATES: 32 G

Mexican-Spiced Tomato and White Bean Soup

Kick things up a notch with this south-of-the-border-inspired soup. Although it is low in calories, each serving has 8 g of protein and almost 7 g of fiber, making it quite filling.

1 (14-OUNCE) CAN LOW-SODIUM GLUTEN-FREE CHICKEN BROTH

2 TEASPOONS CHILI POWDER

1 TEASPOON GROUND CUMIN

1 (16-OUNCE) CAN SODIUM-FREE WHITE BEANS, DRAINED AND RINSED

1 POBLANO CHILE, HALVED AND SEEDED

½ ONION, CUT INTO ½-INCH-THICK WEDGES

1 PINT GRAPE TOMATOES

¼ CUP CHOPPED FRESH CILANTRO

2 TABLESPOONS FRESHLY SQUEEZED LIME JUICE

1 TABLESPOON OLIVE OIL

½ TEASPOON SEA SALT

1. In a Dutch oven or a large stockpot over medium-high heat, combine 1 cup of broth, chili powder, cumin, and beans.

2. In a food processor or blender, combine the remaining broth, poblano chile, and onion. Pulse until the vegetables are coarsely chopped. Add the onion mixture to the Dutch oven.

3. Using the food processor, coarsely chop the tomatoes. Add the tomatoes and cilantro to the Dutch oven.

4. Bring the soup to a boil, cover, and reduce the heat. Simmer the soup for 5 minutes, or until the vegetables are tender.

5. Remove the soup from the heat. Stir in the lime juice, olive oil, and salt.

CALORIES: 157   TOTAL FAT: 4 G   SATURATED FAT: 1 G   SUGAR: 1 G   CARBOHYDRATES: 23 G

Chicken and Sweet Potato Soup with Collard Greens

The ideal antidote to a winter's day, this creamy dish will warm your heart and soul. The combination of ginger, lime, and almond butter also gives the soup a subtle Thai flavor, which will keep things interesting for your taste buds.

4 CUPS LOW-SODIUM GLUTEN-FREE
    CHICKEN STOCK
½ ONION, DICED
1 GARLIC CLOVE, MINCED
1 SWEET POTATO, PEELED AND DICED
8 OUNCES BONELESS, SKINLESS
    CHICKEN BREAST, CUT INTO
    1-INCH PIECES

½ CUP NO-SUGAR-ADDED
    ALMOND BUTTER
1 CUP COLLARD GREENS,
    COARSELY CHOPPED
2 TABLESPOONS MINCED
    FRESH GINGER
SEA SALT
FRESHLY GROUND BLACK PEPPER
1 LIME, QUARTERED

1. In a large stockpot or a Dutch oven, combine the stock, onion, garlic, and sweet potato. Bring the mixture to a boil. Reduce the heat to a simmer, add the chicken, and cover. Simmer for 20 minutes.

2. In a small mixing bowl, whisk together the almond butter and ½ cup of soup from the pot until a thick paste forms. Set aside.

3. Stir the collard greens and ginger into the soup. Bring it back to a boil. Reduce the heat and simmer again, covered, for 5 minutes.

4. Fold in the almond butter paste. Season the soup with salt and pepper.

5. Divide the soup among 4 bowls and squeeze a lime wedge into each.

CALORIES: 353   TOTAL FAT: 21 G   SATURATED FAT: 2 G   SUGAR: 5 G   CARBOHYDRATES: 19 G

Beef and Vegetable Stew

Your diet may be limited, but you can still enjoy thoughtfully prepared comfort foods. If you have a hankering for meat and potatoes, indulge in this one-pot meal, minus the starchy spuds. Although the flavor develops fairly quickly as it cooks, the dish will only taste better the next day.

1 POUND BEEF TENDERLOIN, TRIMMED AND CUT INTO ¼-INCH CUBES

6 CUPS LOW-SODIUM GLUTEN-FREE CHICKEN BROTH

2 CARROTS, PEELED AND CHOPPED

1 RUTABAGA, PEELED AND CHOPPED

2 PARSNIPS, PEELED AND CHOPPED

1 LEEK, WHITE PART ONLY, QUARTERED

2 CELERY STALKS, CHOPPED

1 SPRIG FRESH THYME

1 SPRIG FRESH ROSEMARY

1 SPRIG FRESH PARSLEY

SEA SALT

FRESHLY GROUND BLACK PEPPER

1. In a large stockpot or a Dutch oven, brown the beef on all sides over medium heat, about 6 minutes.

2. Pour in the chicken broth and add the carrots, rutabaga, parsnips, leek, celery, thyme, rosemary, and parsley. Season with salt and pepper. Bring the stew to a boil, reduce the heat, and simmer for 25 minutes, or until the vegetables are tender.

3. Divide the stew among 4 bowls. Serve hot.

CALORIES: 288   TOTAL FAT: 9 G   SATURATED FAT: 3 G   SUGAR: 8 G   CARBOHYDRATES: 23 G

Broiled Vegetable Wraps

The vegetables that make up the sandwich filling in this recipe can also be grilled if you have a barbeque. Just toss all the vegetables in olive oil and season them with sea salt and freshly ground black pepper before grilling them over medium heat until they are lightly charred and tender.

½ EGGPLANT, CUT INTO ½-INCH SLICES
1 ZUCCHINI, CUT LENGTHWISE INTO
    ½-INCH SLICES
1 RED ONION, CUT INTO ½-INCH SLICES
2 TABLESPOONS OLIVE OIL

SEA SALT
FRESHLY GROUND BLACK PEPPER
1 CUP HALVED CHERRY TOMATOES
1 TABLESPOON CHOPPED BASIL
4 (8-INCH) BROWN-RICE TORTILLAS

1. Preheat the oven to broil.

2. Cover a baking sheet with foil.

3. Spread the eggplant, zucchini, and onion on the baking sheet and drizzle them with the olive oil.

4. Season the vegetables with salt and pepper.

5. Broil the vegetables until tender, about 15 minutes, turning once halfway through.

6. Transfer the vegetables to a medium bowl and add the tomatoes and basil. Toss to combine the mixture.

7. Divide the broiled vegetables between the 4 tortillas.

8. Roll up each tortilla and serve 2 per person.

CALORIES: 499   TOTAL FAT: 20 G   SATURATED FAT: 2 G   SUGAR: 7 G   CARBOHYDRATES: 73 G

Ground Lamb and Lentil Lettuce Wraps

Get a taste of the Mediterranean with this flavorful dish. If you don't want to buy all the spices that this recipe calls for, no problem; it will still be delicious if prepared with only cumin and cinnamon to season it.

2 TABLESPOONS OLIVE OIL, PLUS
    ADDITIONAL IF NEEDED
1 POUND FRESHLY GROUND LAMB
1 ONION, DICED
2 GARLIC CLOVES, MINCED
1 TEASPOON GROUND CUMIN
½ TEASPOON GROUND CORIANDER
¼ TEASPOON GROUND CLOVES
¼ TEASPOON GROUND CARDAMOM

½ TEASPOON CINNAMON
1 CUP COOKED LENTILS
6 TABLESPOONS SLICED ALMONDS
PINCH TURMERIC
SEA SALT
FRESHLY GROUND BLACK PEPPER
¼ CUP CHOPPED FRESH CILANTRO
BUTTER LETTUCE LEAVES

1. In a large skillet or a Dutch oven, heat the olive oil over medium heat. Brown the lamb and drain some of the fat from pan, leaving about 1 teaspoon of fat in the pan.

2. Stir in the onion and garlic (add a little olive oil to the pan, if necessary). Add the cumin, coriander, cloves, cardamom, and cinnamon. Stir until all the ingredients and spices are well combined and cook for 3 minutes.

3. Stir in the cooked lentils, almonds, and turmeric. Season with salt and pepper.

4. Remove the Dutch oven from the heat and stir in the cilantro.

5. Divide the lentil mixture among 4 plates. Serve the butter lettuce leaves on the side of each plate, and let your guests spoon the lentils onto each leaf, wrap, and enjoy.

CALORIES: 502   TOTAL FAT: 39 G   SATURATED FAT: 13 G   SUGAR: 1 G   CARBOHYDRATES: 12 G

Pesto Chicken Lettuce Rolls

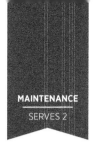

Lettuce makes a fresh wrapping for any filling and does not detract from the flavor of the ingredients. There are many types of lettuce that can be used for your wraps, such as romaine, Boston, or Bibb as well as radicchio and chard. Make sure you trim out any thick cores on the leaves, or the wrapping can crack when you roll it.

3 TABLESPOONS HOMEMADE BLENDER
    MAYONNAISE (PAGE 30)
½ TEASPOON MINCED GARLIC
1 TABLESPOON CHOPPED FRESH BASIL
1 CUP COOKED, CHOPPED
    CHICKEN BREAST
1 CELERY STALK, FINELY DICED

SEA SALT
FRESHLY GROUND BLACK PEPPER
4 BOSTON LETTUCE LEAVES
1 CARROT, PEELED AND SHREDDED
½ CUCUMBER, SHREDDED AND THE
    LIQUID SQUEEZED OUT

1. In a small bowl, combine the mayonnaise, garlic, and basil and stir to mix well.

2. Add the chicken breast and celery to the mayonnaise mixture and stir to combine.

3. Season the mixture with salt and pepper.

4. Spoon the chicken salad evenly into the lettuce leaves.

5. Top the chicken salad with the shredded carrot and cucumber.

6. Roll the lettuce around the chicken filling and serve 2 rolls per person.

CALORIES: 132   TOTAL FAT: 8 G   SATURATED FAT: 1 G   SUGAR: 4 G   CARBOHYDRATES: 13 G

Greek-Style Steak Sandwiches

It is important to marinate your flank steak for the recommended time, because this cut of beef can be tough if not prepared correctly. The acid in the marinade tenderizes the meat and adds a tasty tang to the finished dish.

1 TABLESPOON APPLE CIDER VINEGAR
2 TABLESPOONS OLIVE OIL
1 TEASPOON MINCED GARLIC
1 TEASPOON CHOPPED
    FRESH OREGANO
1 TEASPOON CHOPPED FRESH THYME

10 OUNCES FLANK STEAK,
    TRIMMED OF FAT
2 (8-INCH) BROWN RICE TORTILLAS
1 CUP SHREDDED LETTUCE
½ RED ONION, THINLY SLICED
1 TOMATO, DICED

1. In a sealable freezer bag, combine the apple cider vinegar, olive oil, garlic, oregano, and thyme, and shake to combine.

2. Add the flank steak to the marinade and seal the bag after pressing out the excess air.

3. Place the bag in the fridge and allow the steak to marinate for at least 2 hours, turning the bag several times.

4. Preheat the oven to broil.

5. Line a baking sheet with foil or place a grill pan on a baking sheet.

6. Take the steak out of the bag and discard the marinade. Place the steak on the baking sheet and broil it for 5 minutes per side, or until desired doneness.

7. Remove the steak from the oven and let it rest at least 10 minutes before slicing it thinly across the grain.

8. Stack the sliced steak into the tortillas and top it with the lettuce, onion, and tomato.

9. Roll up the tortillas and serve.

CALORIES: 455 TOTAL FAT: 17 G SATURATED FAT: 5 G SUGAR: 3 G CARBOHYDRATES: 30 G

NOTES

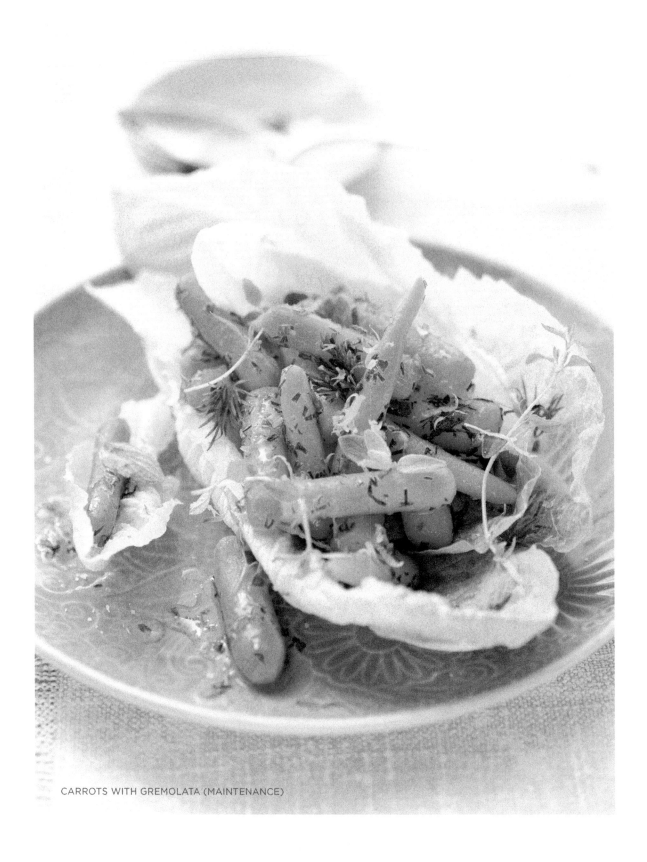

CARROTS WITH GREMOLATA (MAINTENANCE)

8

Salads

CLEANSE

KALE SALAD WITH TOASTED WALNUTS AND EGGS

CHILI-LIME JICAMA WITH DICED CUCUMBERS

QUINOA WITH FRESH HERB VINAIGRETTE

POACHED SALMON AND AVOCADO SALAD

GRILLED CHICKEN AND ARUGULA SALAD

AVOCADO-BASIL CHICKEN SALAD

GRILLED SKIRT STEAK ARUGULA SALAD WITH CILANTRO-LIME VINAIGRETTE

MAINTENANCE

CARROTS WITH GREMOLATA

QUINOA SALAD WITH ROASTED SWEET POTATOES AND APPLES

TRADITIONAL CABBAGE SLAW

EASY BEAN SALAD

PASTEL SPRING SALAD

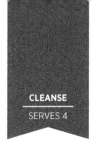
Kale Salad with Toasted Walnuts and Eggs

Eggs are not just for breakfast. They are a great way to bulk up salads with protein. This recipe calls for hard-boiled eggs, but if you like a runny yolk, soft-boiled eggs would work well with the lemony dressing on this dish.

½ TEASPOON GROUND CUMIN

¼ TEASPOON CRUSHED RED PEPPER FLAKES

3 ANCHOVY FILLETS PACKED IN OIL, DRAINED

1 GARLIC CLOVE, MINCED

4 TABLESPOONS FRESHLY SQUEEZED LEMON JUICE

⅓ CUP OLIVE OIL, PLUS MORE FOR DRIZZLING

SEA SALT

FRESHLY GROUND BLACK PEPPER

2 BUNCHES TUSCAN KALE, CENTER RIBS DISCARDED, THINLY SLICED

1 CUP TOASTED WALNUTS

4 HARD-BOILED EGGS, PEELED AND QUARTERED

1. In a food processor, combine the cumin, red pepper flakes, anchovies, and garlic and process until smooth. Whisk in the lemon juice and olive oil, and season with salt and pepper.

2. In a large mixing bowl, toss the kale with the anchovy dressing until well combined. Season the salad with salt and pepper and divide the salad among 4 plates.

3. Top each salad with walnuts, a drizzle of olive oil, and a dash of pepper. Serve the eggs alongside the salad.

CALORIES: 482   TOTAL FAT: 45 G   SATURATED FAT: 8 G   SUGAR: 1 G   CARBOHYDRATES: 12 G

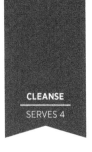

Chili-Lime Jicama with Diced Cucumbers

Sweet and delicate, jicama is a great low-calorie option if you have a need for something crunchy. As a bonus, it's also a good source of fiber and vitamin C. Yummy year-round, this dish can be a refreshing summer salad or a cool pick to complement something spicy. The flavor will develop as the salad sits, so prep it and be patient.

2 TABLESPOONS FRESHLY SQUEEZED
   LIME JUICE
⅛ TEASPOON CHILI POWDER
1 JICAMA, PEELED AND CUT INTO
   ½-INCH CUBES

1 CUCUMBER, PEELED, SEEDED, AND
   CUT INTO ½-INCH CUBES
½ TEASPOON SEA SALT
PINCH CAYENNE PEPPER

1. In a large mixing bowl, combine the lime juice, chili powder, jicama, cucumber, salt, and cayenne pepper. Toss until well combined.

2. Cover and refrigerate the recipe for at least 1 hour before serving.

CALORIES: 70   TOTAL FAT: 0 G   SATURATED FAT: 0 G   SUGAR: 4 G   CARBOHYDRATES: 17 G

Quinoa with Fresh Herb Vinaigrette

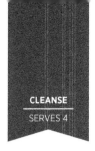

CLEANSE
SERVES 4

Quinoa, a gluten-free grain, is packed with protein and safe to eat on a candida diet. Make sure to rinse it before cooking, since it has an indigestible bitter coating that needs to be washed off.

FOR THE QUINOA

2¾ CUPS LOW-SODIUM GLUTEN-FREE CHICKEN BROTH

¼ CUP FRESHLY SQUEEZED LEMON JUICE

1½ CUPS UNCOOKED QUINOA

FOR THE DRESSING

¼ CUP OLIVE OIL

¼ CUP FRESHLY SQUEEZED LEMON JUICE

¾ CUP CHOPPED FRESH BASIL

¼ CUP CHOPPED FRESH PARSLEY

1 TABLESPOON CHOPPED FRESH THYME

2 TEASPOONS GRATED LEMON ZEST

SEA SALT

FRESHLY GROUND BLACK PEPPER

To make the quinoa:

1. In a medium saucepan over medium-high heat, combine the chicken broth, lemon juice, and quinoa.

2. Bring the mixture to a boil, then reduce the heat to a simmer, cover, and cook until all the liquid is absorbed, 12 to 15 minutes. Let the quinoa cool to room temperature before adding the dressing.

To make the dressing:

1. In a small bowl, mix together the olive oil, lemon juice, basil, parsley, thyme, and lemon zest. Season the mixture with salt and pepper.

2. Pour the dressing over the quinoa, toss to combine, and season it again with salt and pepper.

CALORIES: 391   TOTAL FAT: 18 G   SATURATED FAT: 3 G   SUGAR: 1 G   CARBOHYDRATES: 46 G

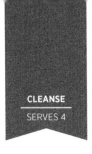

Poached Salmon and Avocado Salad

Omega-3-packed salmon and avocado are a delicious and nutritious power couple that will give your body a heart-healthy fix. Poaching is the suggested method for cooking the salmon, but feel free to broil or grill it. No matter how you choose to prepare the fish, make sure it has cooled before it's folded in with the rest of the salad ingredients. The salad can stand alone or be served on a bed of fresh spinach or crispy romaine lettuce, with a side of lemon wedges for an extra splash of citrus.

2 CARROTS, PEELED AND HALVED

1 CELERY STALK, HALVED

1 ONION, HALVED

½ LEMON, HALVED

6 CUPS WATER

1 POUND WILD SALMON FILLET, SKIN REMOVED

SEA SALT

1 AVOCADO, PEELED, PITTED, AND CUBED

½ RED ONION, THINLY SLICED

2 TABLESPOONS FRESHLY SQUEEZED LEMON JUICE

2 TABLESPOONS OLIVE OIL

1 TABLESPOON CHOPPED FRESH DILL

1 TABLESPOON CHOPPED FRESH CHIVES

FRESHLY GROUND BLACK PEPPER

1. In a Dutch oven or a stockpot, combine the carrots, celery, onion, lemon, and water. Bring the mixture to a boil, then reduce the heat to medium-low, cover, and cook for 8 minutes.

2. Season the salmon with a pinch of salt. Gently place the fish in the broth mixture. Reduce the heat to a simmer, cover, and cook until the salmon is opaque, about 5 minutes. Using a slotted spoon, remove the salmon from the liquid.

3. In a large mixing bowl, flake the salmon into chunks using a fork. Refrigerate the salmon in the bowl until it has cooled, 20 to 30 minutes.

4. When the salmon has cooled, fold in the avocado, red onion, lemon juice, olive oil, dill, and chives. Season the mixture with salt and pepper. Refrigerate the salad for at least 30 minutes to allow the flavors to blend.

CALORIES: 356   TOTAL FAT: 24 G   SATURATED FAT: 4 G   SUGAR: 6 G   CARBOHYDRATES: 6 G

Grilled Chicken and Arugula Salad

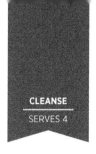

Don't take greens for granted! You may be used to covering them with salad dressings, but each variety has a distinct flavor that becomes even more pronounced when eaten fresh. Peppery arugula is showcased in this dish, and complemented beautifully by a simple seasoned splash of lemon and olive oil. Grilling the chicken will add flavor to the lean cut, but you may also panfry them in a heavy skillet with just a splash of oil.

4 (6-OUNCE) BONELESS, SKINLESS
   CHICKEN BREASTS
½ TEASPOON GROUND CORIANDER
SEA SALT
FRESHLY GROUND BLACK PEPPER
3 TABLESPOONS OLIVE OIL

3 TABLESPOONS FRESHLY SQUEEZED
   LEMON JUICE
5 OUNCES (ABOUT 6 CUPS) BABY
   ARUGULA
4 RADISHES, THINLY SLICED
½ RED ONION, THINLY SLICED

1. Heat the grill to high.

2. Without cutting all the way through, split each chicken breast in half horizontally to butterfly it. Place the breasts in a large plastic freezer bag or in between 2 sheets of wax paper. Using a meat mallet, pound out the breasts until they are about ½-inch thick.

3. Season each breast with coriander, salt, and pepper.

4. Grill or panfry the breasts for 2 or 3 minutes per side, or until cooked through.

5. In a large mixing bowl, whisk together the oil, lemon juice, and a pinch of salt and pepper. Toss in the arugula, radishes, and onion. Mix until the ingredients are well combined.

6. Divide the salad between 4 plates. Top each serving with a grilled chicken breast.

CALORIES: 289   TOTAL FAT: 14 G   SATURATED FAT: 3 G   SUGAR: 1 G   CARBOHYDRATES: 3 G

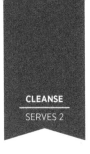

Avocado-Basil Chicken Salad

There's no need for mayonnaise in this chicken salad, thanks to the creaminess of the avocados. The fresh basil will give this dish a bright flavor that may be amped up even more with a squeeze of lime. You can serve this dish as a sandwich on Almond Butter Bread (page 128), or on a bed of crispy romaine lettuce.

1 AVOCADO, PEELED, PITTED, AND HALVED

½ CUP BASIL LEAVES, STEMS REMOVED AND DISCARDED

2 TABLESPOONS OLIVE OIL

½ TEASPOON SEA SALT

⅛ TEASPOON FRESHLY GROUND BLACK PEPPER

2 (6-OUNCE) BONELESS, SKINLESS CHICKEN BREASTS, COOKED AND SHREDDED

1. Place the avocado in a food processor or blender. Add in the basil, olive oil, salt, and black pepper, and combine until smooth.

2. Pour the mixture into a large mixing bowl. Add the shredded chicken and toss until well combined. Season with salt and pepper.

3. Refrigerate the chicken salad for about 15 minutes before serving.

CALORIES: 506   TOTAL FAT: 19 G   SATURATED FAT: 3 G   SUGAR: 0 G   CARBOHYDRATES: 0 G

Grilled Skirt Steak Arugula Salad with Cilantro-Lime Vinaigrette

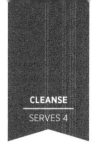

Although there seem to be a lot of ingredients in this dish, there aren't many steps in preparing it, and it comes together fairly quickly. Thanks to the flavorful dressing, there's really no need to marinate the meat before cooking.

FOR THE DRESSING

⅓ CUP OLIVE OIL

¼ CUP FRESHLY SQUEEZED LIME JUICE

½ CUP PACKED FRESH
    CILANTRO LEAVES

½ TEASPOON SEA SALT

½ JALAPEÑO PEPPER, SEEDED

1 GARLIC CLOVE

FOR THE STEAK

1 POUND SKIRT STEAK

1 TABLESPOON SEA SALT

1 TABLESPOON OLIVE OIL

FRESHLY GROUND BLACK PEPPER

FOR THE SALAD

1 BUNCH ARUGULA

½ PINT GRAPE TOMATOES, HALVED

1 AVOCADO, PEELED, PITTED,
    AND DICED

½ RED ONION, THINLY SLICED

To make the dressing:

1. In a blender, combine all ingredients and pulse until the solids are well chopped. Set aside.

To make the steak:

1. Preheat a grill or heat a grill pan to high.

2. Season the steak with salt and set aside for 5 minutes.

3. Brush both sides of the steak with olive oil and season with black pepper.

continued ▶

4. Grill the steak for 3 to 5 minutes per side.

5. Remove the steak from the heat and let it rest for 10 minutes. Slice the steak against the grain into ¼-inch strips.

To make the salad:

1. On a large platter, arrange an even layer of arugula. Top it with the sliced skirt steak, then scatter tomatoes, avocado chunks, and red onion slices around the salad. Drizzle the salad with the cilantro-lime dressing.

CALORIES: 524   TOTAL FAT: 42 G   SATURATED FAT: 9 G   SUGAR: 2 G   CARBOHYDRATES: 8 G

Carrots with Gremolata

Gremolata is a fancy word for a sauce made of chopped herbs and lemon zest. The sauce can be used on vegetables, as it is here, or served alongside meat or fish.

1½ POUNDS CARROTS, PEELED AND
    CUT ON THE DIAGONAL INTO
    3-INCH-LONG PIECES, HALVED
    LENGTHWISE
½ CUP LOW-SODIUM GLUTEN-FREE
    CHICKEN BROTH
4 TEASPOONS OLIVE OIL

SEA SALT
FRESHLY GROUND BLACK PEPPER
¼ CUP CHOPPED FRESH MINT
¼ CUP CHOPPED FRESH PARSLEY
2 TEASPOONS FRESHLY SQUEEZED
    LEMON JUICE
½ TEASPOON GRATED LEMON ZEST

1. In a large skillet over medium-high heat, combine the carrots, broth, and 1 teaspoon of oil. Bring the mixture to a boil, cover, reduce the heat to medium, and cook until the carrots are tender, 12 to 14 minutes.

2. Uncover and cook, stirring, until the liquid has evaporated and the carrots are lightly browned, 2 to 3 more minutes. Season with salt and pepper.

3. In a small bowl, combine the mint, parsley, lemon juice, lemon zest, and remaining 3 teaspoons of oil. Season the gremolata with salt and pepper.

4. Toss the carrots with the herb mixture and serve.

———————

CALORIES: 110   TOTAL FAT: 5 G   SATURATED FAT: 1 G   SUGAR: 8 G   CARBOHYDRATES: 17 G

Quinoa Salad with Roasted Sweet Potatoes and Apples

Between roasting the sweet potatoes and cooking the quinoa, the prep time for this salad may be a little much. To save time, cook these components the day before you need them; they are still fresh and delicious if served within a few days.

8 TABLESPOONS OLIVE OIL

1½ CUPS UNCOOKED QUINOA

3 CUPS WATER

SEA SALT

1½ POUNDS SWEET POTATOES, PEELED AND DICED INTO ¾-INCH CUBES

FRESHLY GROUND BLACK PEPPER

¼ CUP APPLE CIDER VINEGAR

2 GRANNY SMITH APPLES, DICED INTO ½-INCH CUBES

½ CUP CHOPPED FRESH FLAT-LEAF PARSLEY

½ RED ONION, THINLY SLICED

6 OUNCES BABY SPINACH

1. Preheat the oven to 400°F.

2. In a large saucepan, heat 1 tablespoon of olive oil over medium heat. Add the quinoa and toast for 2 minutes, stirring constantly so it doesn't burn.

3. Pour in the water, add a pinch of salt, and bring the water to a boil. Reduce the heat to a simmer, cover, and cook the quinoa for 15 minutes. Remove the saucepan from the heat, let it stand for 10 minutes, then fluff it with a fork. Transfer the quinoa to a bowl and refrigerate it until it's chilled, about 20 minutes.

4. In a large mixing bowl, toss the sweet potatoes with 1 tablespoon of olive oil. Season the sweet potatoes with salt and pepper. Spread the sweet potatoes on a baking sheet and roast them until tender, about 25 minutes, stirring halfway. Remove the baking sheet from the heat and allow the sweet potatoes to cool.

5. In a large mixing bowl, whisk together the remaining 6 tablespoons of olive oil and vinegar. Season the mixture with salt and pepper.

6. Stir in the cooked quinoa, roasted sweet potatoes, apples, parsley, onion, and spinach. Toss until everything is well combined. Serve immediately.

CALORIES: 283   TOTAL FAT: 12 G   SATURATED FAT: 2 G   SUGAR: 5 G   CARBOHYDRATES: 41 G

Traditional Cabbage Slaw

Coleslaw is perfect comfort food, and the taste gets better if it is allowed to mellow, so make a double recipe and enjoy it for several days. You can also add grated broccoli, asparagus, and chopped kale to the mix for texture and a nice assertive flavor.

½ HEAD RED CABBAGE, SHREDDED

½ HEAD GREEN CABBAGE, SHREDDED

2 CARROTS, PEELED AND SHREDDED

½ RED ONION, PEELED AND
    THINLY SLICED

¾ CUP HOMEMADE BLENDER
    MAYONNAISE (PAGE 30)

2 TABLESPOONS APPLE CIDER
    VINEGAR

¼ TEASPOON LIQUID STEVIA

SEA SALT

FRESHLY GROUND BLACK PEPPER

1. In a large bowl, toss together the cabbages, carrots, and onion.

2. In a small bowl, whisk together the mayonnaise, vinegar, and stevia until they are well blended.

3. Toss the cabbage mixture with the dressing until coated.

4. Season the slaw with salt and pepper.

5. Place the slaw in the fridge for at least 30 minutes to let the cabbage soften before serving.

CALORIES: 236   TOTAL FAT: 15 G   SATURATED FAT: 2 G   SUGAR: 11 G   CARBOHYDRATES: 25 G

Easy Bean Salad

There are many healthy canned bean options in grocery stores, but if you have time, you can also cook your beans from dry. Use one cup of each bean and make sure you pick through them well for grit and stones. Cook your beans according to the package instructions and allow them to cool completely before tossing this salad together.

2 CUPS FRESH GREEN BEANS, CUT INTO 1-INCH PIECES

1 (16-OUNCE) CAN SODIUM-FREE KIDNEY BEANS, DRAINED AND RINSED

1 (16-OUNCE) CAN SODIUM-FREE PINTO BEANS, DRAINED AND RINSED

1 (16-OUNCE) CAN SODIUM-FREE NAVY BEANS, DRAINED AND RINSED

1 (16-OUNCE) CAN SODIUM-FREE CHICKPEAS, DRAINED AND RINSED

1 RED ONION, PEELED AND THINLY SLICED

½ CUP OLIVE OIL

½ CUP APPLE CIDER VINEGAR

1 TEASPOON MINCED GARLIC

1 TEASPOON DRY MUSTARD

1 TEASPOON CHOPPED FRESH THYME

PINCH STEVIA

SEA SALT

FRESHLY GROUND BLACK PEPPER

1. In a large bowl, combine the green beans, kidney beans, pinto beans, navy beans, chickpeas, and onion until they are well mixed.

2. In a small bowl, whisk together the olive oil, apple cider vinegar, garlic, mustard, thyme, and stevia until blended.

3. Toss the dressing with the beans.

4. Season the beans with salt and pepper.

5. Let the salad chill in the fridge for at least 1 hour to allow the flavors to mellow.

CALORIES: 404   TOTAL FAT: 18 G   SATURATED FAT: 3 G   SUGAR: 4 G   CARBOHYDRATES: 48 G

Pastel Spring Salad

This dish is stunning to look at, impressive enough for a fancy restaurant, but enjoyed in the comforts of your home. You get many different textures and colors in each bite, which ensures you're getting a broad range of nutrients to keep your body healthy. There is no dressing in this recipe, but a light herb vinaigrette can be used if you want a little more taste.

4 CUPS SHREDDED SPINACH

1 CUCUMBER, DICED

3 RADISHES, THINLY SLICED

2 TANGERINES, PEELED AND
    SEGMENTED

1 CUP SNAP PEAS, STRINGED AND
    SNIPPED IN HALF

1 CUP HALVED CHERRY TOMATOES

2 TABLESPOONS FRESH
    CHOPPED MINT

JUICE OF 1 LEMON

4 TABLESPOONS CHOPPED ALMONDS

SEA SALT

FRESHLY GROUND BLACK PEPPER

1. Arrange the spinach on 2 plates.

2. Layered on top of the spinach, evenly divide the cucumber, radishes, tangerine segments, peas, and cherry tomatoes.

3. Sprinkle each salad with mint, lemon juice, and almonds.

4. Season the salads with salt and pepper. Serve immediately.

CALORIES: 228   TOTAL FAT: 7 G   SATURATED FAT: 1 G   SUGAR: 16 G   CARBOHYDRATES: 36 G

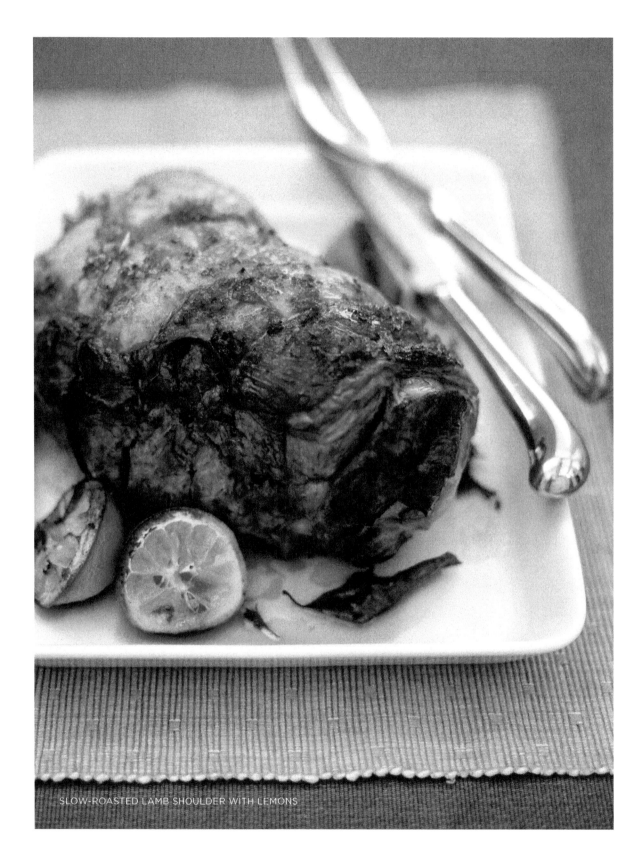

SLOW-ROASTED LAMB SHOULDER WITH LEMONS

9

Main Dishes

CLEANSE

LENTIL CURRY WITH SPINACH

VEGETABLE "FRIED RICE"

VEGETABLE NASI GORENG

RAW PAD THAI

SALMON WITH GARLIC AND GINGER

GRILLED MOROCCAN SALMON

POACHED SALMON WITH WARM TOMATOES

PAN-SEARED HERRING WITH LIME AND PEPPER

LIME-GARLIC CHICKEN WITH AVOCADO SALSA

COCONUT CHICKEN WITH BOK CHOY

SPICY CHICKEN PATTIES

GARLIC AND ROSEMARY CHICKEN THIGHS

ZUCCHINI "SPAGHETTI" WITH CHICKEN

KID-FRIENDLY CHICKEN FINGERS

HERB-ROASTED TURKEY TENDERLOIN

LAMB VINDALOO

SLOW-ROASTED LAMB SHOULDER WITH LEMONS

GRILLED BEEF SKEWERS WITH ZUCCHINI

GRILLED SIRLOIN WITH GARLIC BUTTER

LEMONY POT ROAST

MAINTENANCE

SWEET POTATO COLCANNON

SPICY VEGETARIAN CHILI

CURRIED QUINOA

ROASTED CHICKEN WITH PEARS

HERBED CHICKEN WITH WHITE BEANS

BROILED LEMON CHICKEN

SAVORY STUFFED TOMATOES WITH TURKEY

TURKEY CABBAGE ROLLS

CHILI TURKEY BURGERS

TRADITIONAL MEATLOAF

Lentil Curry with Spinach

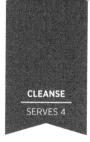

Indian food is perfect for those who suffer from candida sensitivity. If you've never cooked with curry leaves before, they are available in Indian grocery stores and have nothing to do with the spice of the same name. If you can't find them, leave them out or substitute bay leaves instead.

2½ CUPS WATER

1⅓ CUPS UNCOOKED YELLOW LENTILS

¼ TEASPOON TURMERIC

¼ TEASPOON SEA SALT

2 TEASPOONS COCONUT OIL

7 GARLIC CLOVES, MINCED

1 TABLESPOON MINCED FRESH GINGER

1 CUP PACKED BABY SPINACH, CHOPPED

3 DRIED MILD RED CHILIES, BROKEN UP BY HAND

1 TEASPOON WHOLE MUSTARD SEEDS

1 TEASPOON WHOLE CUMIN SEEDS

6 CURRY LEAVES

2 TABLESPOONS CHOPPED FRESH CILANTRO

2 TABLESPOONS FRESHLY SQUEEZED LEMON JUICE

1. In a medium saucepan, combine the water, lentils, turmeric, and salt. Bring the mixture to a boil over high heat, then reduce the heat to low. Cover and cook for 25 minutes or until the lentils are soft.

2. Strain the lentils, reserving ¼ cup of cooking water. Return the lentils and the reserved cooking water to the saucepan, mash lightly, and set aside.

3. In a separate pan over medium heat, sauté 1 teaspoon of coconut oil, 4 minced garlic cloves, and ginger for 1 minute.

4. Add the spinach and cook for 2 minutes, or until the spinach is lightly wilted. Add the spinach mixture to the lentils.

5. In the same saucepan the spinach cooked in, add the remaining 1 teaspoon of coconut oil, remaining 3 garlic cloves, red chilies, mustard seeds, cumin seeds, and curry leaves. Heat the mixture on medium-high until the seeds begin to pop and turn golden.

6. Add the spices to the lentil mixture and stir to combine. Cook the entire dish in the saucepan for 5 to 10 more minutes, then stir in the cilantro and lemon juice. Serve warm.

CALORIES: 418   TOTAL FAT: 11 G   SATURATED FAT: 2 G   SUGAR: 0 G   CARBOHYDRATES: 4 G

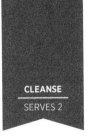
Vegetable "Fried Rice"

The "rice" in this dish is actually cauliflower that's been pulsed in a food processor. With all the traditional flavors of take-out Chinese, you'll never miss the grain.

6 CUPS CAULIFLOWER FLORETS

2 GARLIC CLOVES, MINCED

2 TABLESPOONS COCONUT OIL

1 CUP CHOPPED CARROTS

2 TABLESPOONS CHOPPED
   GREEN ONION

2 EGGS, BEATEN

TAMARI (GLUTEN-FREE SOY SAUCE)

SEA SALT

1. Put the cauliflower in a food processor and pulse until it resembles rice.

2. In a large skillet over medium heat, sauté the garlic in the coconut oil.

3. Add the carrots and a splash of water to prevent the vegetables from sticking, and cook for 5 minutes, or until the carrots are crisp-tender.

4. Add the green onion and eggs and cook for 30 seconds.

5. Add in the cauliflower "rice" along with a splash of tamari and salt. Stir to combine and cook for 3 to 5 minutes, or until the mixture is heated through and the eggs are cooked.

CALORIES: 302   TOTAL FAT: 20 G   SATURATED FAT: 14 G   SUGAR: 4 G   CARBOHYDRATES: 24 G

Vegetable Nasi Goreng

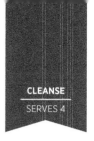
Nasi Goreng is a traditional Indonesian dish that usually features shrimp, pork, or chicken along with the fried-rice base. This vegetarian version is just as satisfying and can be eaten cold the next day for lunch because the flavors intensify over time. You can kick up the heat by adding an additional chile pepper if you like spicy food.

3 EGGS

1 TEASPOON BUTTER

3 TABLESPOONS SESAME OIL

1 SWEET ONION, PEELED AND DICED

1 LEEK, DICED

2 TEASPOONS MINCED GARLIC

1 CHILE PEPPER, MINCED

2 CARROTS, PEELED AND DICED

3 CUPS COOKED BROWN RICE

1 TEASPOON GROUND CUMIN

1 TEASPOON GROUND CORIANDER

¼ TEASPOON GROUND GINGER

1 GREEN ONION, THINLY SLICED

2 TABLESPOONS CHOPPED
     FRESH CILANTRO

SEA SALT

1. Place a small skillet over medium-high heat and scramble the eggs in the butter until they are cooked but still slightly moist, about 3 minutes. Set aside.

2. Place a large skillet or wok over medium-high heat and add the sesame oil.

3. Sauté the onion, leek, garlic, and chile in the sesame oil until softened, about 3 minutes.

4. Add the carrot and sauté the mixture for 2 more minutes.

5. Stir in the rice, cumin, coriander, and ginger, and sauté the mixture for 4 to 5 minutes or until the rice is heated through.

6. Remove the skillet from the heat and stir in the eggs, green onion, and cilantro.

7. Season the mixture with salt and serve.

CALORIES: 476   TOTAL FAT: 13 G   SATURATED FAT: 3 G   SUGAR: 3 G   CARBOHYDRATES: 79 G

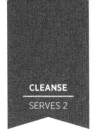

Raw Pad Thai

Raw food can be a valuable source for recipes that are compatible with the candida diet. As long as the ingredients are on the approved list, you can experiment with this fresh, flavor-packed cuisine. The noodles in this dish are replaced with long strips of vegetables, and the peanut sauce is replaced with an almond-based variation. The results are incredibly flavorful and gorgeous to look at on your plate.

JUICE OF 1 LIME

2 TABLESPOONS ALMOND BUTTER

1 TEASPOON TAMARI (OPTIONAL)

½ JALAPEÑO PEPPER, CHOPPED

1 TEASPOON MINCED GARLIC

2 CARROTS, SHREDDED

1 ZUCCHINI, SHREDDED

2 CUPS SHREDDED RED CABBAGE

2 CUPS BEAN SPROUTS

4 GREEN ONIONS, THINLY SLICED

¼ CUP CHOPPED FRESH CILANTRO

1. In a small bowl, combine the lime juice, almond butter, tamari (if using), jalapeño, and garlic until they are well blended.

2. In a large bowl, toss together the carrots, zucchini, cabbage, bean sprouts, onions, and cilantro.

3. Toss the dressing with the vegetables.

4. Let the mixture sit for at least 30 minutes in the fridge to allow the flavors to mellow before serving.

CALORIES: 232   TOTAL FAT: 10 G   SATURATED FAT: 1 G   SUGAR: 9 G   CARBOHYDRATES: 26 G

Salmon with Garlic and Ginger

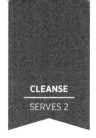

CLEANSE
SERVES 2

Salmon is full of omega-3 fatty acids, which have been shown to improve heart health. Wild salmon is more expensive, but it is the best and cleanest choice, so go ahead and splurge.

2 TABLESPOONS MINCED GARLIC

2 TABLESPOONS GRATED
    FRESH GINGER

2 TEASPOONS COCONUT OIL

½ TEASPOON SEA SALT

FRESHLY GROUND BLACK PEPPER

2 (6-OUNCE) WILD SALMON FILLETS

1. Preheat the broiler to high.

2. In a small bowl, combine the garlic, ginger, coconut oil, salt, and pepper. Spread the mixture over the salmon and set it in a baking pan.

3. Broil the salmon close to the broiler for 2 to 3 minutes. When the crust begins to turn brown, turn the broiler off and set the oven to 300°F.

4. Reposition the salmon into the middle of the oven and bake it until the fish is opaque throughout and flakes with a fork, about 10 minutes.

CALORIES: 291   TOTAL FAT: 16 G   SATURATED FAT: 6 G   SUGAR: 0 G   CARBOHYDRATES: 2 G

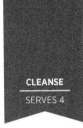

Grilled Moroccan Salmon

The combination of cinnamon with spices makes a palate-pleasing dish. Serve this with grilled asparagus or a spinach salad.

¼ TEASPOON CINNAMON

1 TEASPOON CURRY POWDER

½ TEASPOON GROUND CORIANDER

½ TEASPOON GROUND CUMIN

½ TEASPOON SEA SALT

½ TEASPOON FRESHLY GROUND
 BLACK PEPPER

4 (6-OUNCE) WILD SALMON FILLETS

1. Preheat the grill to medium-high heat, or heat a heavy cast-iron skillet on the stovetop to high heat.

2. In a small bowl, combine the cinnamon, curry powder, coriander, cumin, salt, and pepper. Rub the spice mixture over the top of the salmon to coat it.

3. Grill the salmon, skin-side down, for 8 to 12 minutes, or until it reaches your desired doneness. Or cook the salmon in the skillet for 10 to 12 minutes, or until done.

CALORIES: 243   TOTAL FAT: 11 G   SATURATED FAT: 2 G   SUGAR: 0 G   CARBOHYDRATES: 1 G

Poached Salmon with Warm Tomatoes

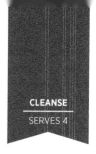

Poaching is the easiest way to cook fish, since it's tough to overcook it that way or dry it out. Poaching also has the added benefit of cutting down on fish aromas in the kitchen.

4 (6-OUNCE) WILD SALMON FILLETS
SEA SALT
FRESHLY GROUND BLACK PEPPER
2 TABLESPOONS UNSALTED BUTTER
1½ CUPS GRAPE TOMATOES

1 BUNCH SCALLIONS, WHITE
   AND LIGHT-GREEN PARTS,
   THINLY SLICED
LEMON WEDGES

1. Fill a large pot with enough water to cover the salmon by at least 1 inch. Bring the water to a simmer.

2. Sprinkle the salmon fillets with salt and pepper on both sides.

3. When the water is simmering, add the salmon. Increase the heat so the water returns to a light simmer, and poach the fish until it is opaque in the center, about 10 minutes for every inch of thickness. Remove the salmon from the water using a large slotted spoon.

4. Heat the butter in a skillet over medium heat until the butter melts and begins to foam. Add the tomatoes to the pan and season them with salt and pepper. Cook the tomatoes for 2 minutes, stirring frequently, then add the scallions. Stir and continue cooking the tomatoes until they begin to wrinkle, about 5 more minutes.

5. Serve the salmon with the tomato mixture and any juices from the skillet, along with the lemon wedges.

CALORIES: 350   TOTAL FAT: 18 G   SATURATED FAT: 6 G   SUGAR: 2 G   CARBOHYDRATES: 5 G

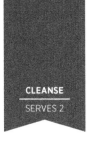

Pan-Seared Herring with Lime and Pepper

Herring is an inexpensive fish that is allowed at all stages of the candida diet. It's full of protein and omega-3 fatty acids, making it a perfect centerpiece for a healthy dinner.

1 ROUNDED TEASPOON WHOLE
    PEPPERCORNS
2 LIMES
1 ROUNDED TABLESPOON
    ALMOND FLOUR

2 (4- TO 5-OUNCE) HERRING FILLETS
2 TABLESPOONS OLIVE OIL
SEA SALT

1. Using a mortar and pestle, crush the peppercorns, making sure they still have some coarseness and texture to them.

2. Zest both limes and add half the zest to the peppercorns.

3. Add the flour to the peppercorn mixture and mix well. Spread the flour mixture on a shallow dish.

4. Dry off the herrings with a paper towel and butterfly, or open, them. Coat the flesh side with the flour mixture, pressing it in well. Dust the skin side with any flour left in the dish.

5. Heat the oil in a large sauté pan over medium-high heat. Fry the herrings, flesh-side down, for 2 to 3 minutes, or until they are golden brown.

6. Turn the fish over and cook them for another 2 minutes. Transfer the fish to paper towels to drain.

7. Season the fish with salt. Serve the herring with the remaining lime zest sprinkled on top and lime wedges on the side.

CALORIES: 414   TOTAL FAT: 32 G   SATURATED FAT: 4 G   SUGAR: 0 G   CARBOHYDRATES: 13 G

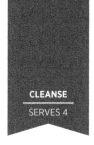
Lime-Garlic Chicken with Avocado Salsa

While you usually want to eat perfectly ripe avocados, the one in this dish should be on the firm side (but still not rock hard). Otherwise the chunks won't hold their shape when you mix up the salsa.

2 GARLIC CLOVES, MINCED

3 TABLESPOONS FRESHLY SQUEEZED
    LIME JUICE

5 TABLESPOONS OLIVE OIL

¼ TEASPOON RED PEPPER FLAKES

SEA SALT

1 POUND BONELESS, SKINLESS
    CHICKEN BREASTS, CUT
    INTO 4 PIECES

1 AVOCADO, PEELED, PITTED,
    AND DICED

¼ CUP CHOPPED RED ONION

2 TABLESPOONS CHOPPED FRESH
    CORIANDER

FRESHLY GROUND BLACK PEPPER

1 LIME, CUT INTO WEDGES

½ CUP SHREDDED CABBAGE

1. In a small bowl, whisk together the garlic, 2 tablespoons of lime juice, 3 tablespoons of olive oil, and red pepper flakes.

2. Season the mixture with salt, then pour it over the chicken and allow it to marinate in the refrigerator for 20 minutes.

3. Place the chicken breasts and marinade in a heavy skillet over high heat. Brown the chicken on both sides and continue cooking until the chicken is cooked through and the juices run clear, 8 to 10 minutes.

4. While the chicken is cooking, mix together the avocado, remaining 1 tablespoon of lime juice, remaining 2 tablespoons of olive oil, red onion, and coriander. Season the mixture with salt and pepper.

5. Serve the chicken topped with the salsa and garnished with lime wedges and cabbage.

CALORIES: 343   TOTAL FAT: 25 G   SATURATED FAT: 4 G   SUGAR: 1 G   CARBOHYDRATES: 7 G

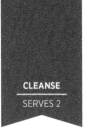
Coconut Chicken with Bok Choy

Coconut aminos is coconut tree sap, and it has a flavor similar to soy sauce. That's what helps give this dish an Asian flavor. If you need a starch to go with this, serve it with quinoa rather than white rice.

1 TEASPOON COCONUT OIL

1 GARLIC CLOVE, THINLY SLICED

3 THIN SLICES FRESH GINGER

1 (12-OUNCE) CAN UNSWEETENED COCONUT MILK

2 TEASPOONS TURMERIC

¼ TEASPOON SEA SALT

3 HEADS BABY BOK CHOY, HALVED LENGTHWISE

4 SCALLIONS, HALVED LENGTHWISE

1 TABLESPOON COCONUT AMINOS

RED PEPPER FLAKES

FRESH BASIL LEAVES

2 SKINLESS, BONELESS CHICKEN BREASTS

1. In a large skillet over medium heat, warm the coconut oil. Add the garlic and ginger, and sauté for 30 seconds.

2. Whisk in the coconut milk, turmeric, and salt, and bring it to a gentle boil.

3. Add the bok choy and scallions, then reduce the heat to medium low. Cover and simmer the mixture for 5 minutes.

4. Stir in the coconut aminos and red pepper flakes, garnish with the fresh basil, and set aside.

5. Heat up a grill to high or a heavy skillet to medium-high and cook the chicken breasts for 5 minutes on each side, or until they are cooked through. Season them with salt and pepper and slice in strips.

6. Divide the bok choy mixture between 2 plates, top the greens with the sliced chicken, and serve.

CALORIES: 330   TOTAL FAT: 22 G   SATURATED FAT: 20 G   SUGAR: 1 G   CARBOHYDRATES: 5 G

Spicy Chicken Patties

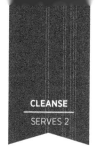

If you're sick of plain chicken breasts, try this flavor-packed dish. The patties are delicious served over sautéed spinach.

8 OUNCES FRESHLY GROUND CHICKEN

2 EGGS

1 TEASPOON ONION POWDER

1 TEASPOON GARLIC POWDER

1 TEASPOON CURRY POWDER

1 TEASPOON DRIED PARSLEY

½ TEASPOON SEA SALT

2 TABLESPOONS COCONUT OIL

1. In a large bowl, mix together the chicken, eggs, onion powder, garlic powder, curry powder, dried parsley, and salt.

2. Put the mixture in the refrigerator for 20 minutes to firm up. Form it into 4 patties.

3. Heat the coconut oil in a sauté pan over medium heat. Put the patties in the pan and cook them for 7 to 8 minutes per side, or until cooked through. Serve two patties per plate.

CALORIES: 374 TOTAL FAT: 30 G SATURATED FAT: 17 G SUGAR: 1 G CARBOHYDRATES: 3 G

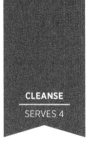

Garlic and Rosemary Chicken Thighs

Most people grab chicken breasts at the meat counter, but thighs are another great option. Get ones on the bone and with skin still attached for this dish, so that you get the most flavor out of the meat.

8 CHICKEN THIGHS, BONE IN AND
    SKIN ON

5 GARLIC CLOVES, MINCED

SEA SALT

FRESHLY GROUND BLACK PEPPER

8 SPRIGS FRESH ROSEMARY

1. Preheat the oven to 350°F.

2. Place the chicken thighs skin-side up in a roasting pan. Scatter the garlic over them and season the garlic and chicken with salt and pepper. Top each chicken thigh with a piece of rosemary.

3. Roast the chicken for 1 hour, or until it is cooked through and the juices run clear. Serve 2 chicken thighs per plate.

CALORIES: 174   TOTAL FAT: 6 G   SATURATED FAT: 2 G   SUGAR: 0 G   CARBOHYDRATES: 2 G

Zucchini "Spaghetti" with Chicken

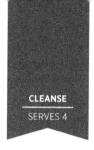
A mandoline slicer is a convenient addition to your kitchen if you use a lot of sliced or julienned vegetables such as the zucchini in this "pasta" dish. A mandolin is a French slicer that uses parallel and perpendicular blades to create sticks, crinkle-cut fries, or julienned vegetables. You can also use a sharp, good-quality kitchen knife if time is not an issue.

6 ZUCCHINI, JULIENNED

¼ TEASPOON SEA SALT

½ TEASPOON BUTTER

2 CUPS CHOPPED COOKED CHICKEN

2 CUPS CHOPPED BROCCOLI

2 GREEN ONIONS, THINLY SLICED

¼ CUP HOMEMADE BASIL PESTO
   (PAGE 34)

3 TABLESPOONS CHOPPED PECANS

1. In a large bowl, combine the zucchini and salt.

2. Let this mixture sit for at least 30 minutes, then carefully squeeze the moisture out of the zucchini.

3. While the zucchini is sitting in the bowl, heat the butter in a large skillet over medium-high heat.

4. Sauté the chicken, broccoli, and green onion until tender, about 5 minutes.

5. Toss the vegetables with the pesto until the vegetables are well coated.

6. Remove the skillet from the heat and add the zucchini.

7. Toss to combine and serve the "spaghetti" topped with the chopped pecans.

CALORIES: 339   TOTAL FAT: 18 G   SATURATED FAT: 3 G   SUGAR: 9 G   CARBOHYDRATES: 19 G

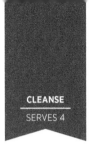

Kid-Friendly Chicken Fingers

You don't need milk and flour (or a deep fryer) to make crispy chicken fingers your whole family will love! Almonds and coconut flour are perfect substitutes.

NONSTICK COOKING SPRAY

2 (8-OUNCE) BONELESS, SKINLESS
   CHICKEN BREASTS

½ CUP SLICED ALMONDS

¼ CUP COCONUT FLOUR

1½ TEASPOONS PAPRIKA

½ TEASPOON GARLIC POWDER

½ TEASPOON DRY MUSTARD

½ TEASPOON SEA SALT

FRESHLY GROUND BLACK PEPPER

1½ TEASPOONS COCONUT OIL

4 EGGS

1. Preheat the oven to 475°F.

2. Line a baking sheet with foil, set a rack over the foil, and coat the rack with cooking spray.

3. Slice the chicken breasts into 1-inch strips.

4. In a food processor, add the almonds, coconut flour, paprika, garlic powder, dry mustard, salt, and pepper. Process until the almonds are finely chopped.

5. Keep the food processor running and slowly drizzle in the coconut oil. Process until well combined, then transfer the mixture to a shallow dish.

6. In a separate shallow dish, whisk the eggs.

7. Dip each chicken strip in the egg mixture, 1 at a time. Hold each strip so the excess drips off, then coat each in the almond mixture.

8. Place the strips on the prepared rack and spray the tops with cooking spray. Turn the chicken fingers over and spray the other side.

9. Bake until the chicken fingers are golden brown and cooked through, 20 to 25 minutes.

CALORIES: 321   TOTAL FAT: 17 G   SATURATED FAT: 7 G   SUGAR: 2 G   CARBOHYDRATES: 7 G

Herb-Roasted Turkey Tenderloin

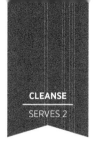

Turkey isn't just for Thanksgiving. Cook up a lean turkey tenderloin for a quick, nutritious dinner any night. Turkey tenderloins are the tender strips of white meat that lay under the turkey breast.

1 TEASPOON DRIED ROSEMARY, CRUSHED

1 TEASPOON DRIED THYME

1 TEASPOON PAPRIKA

1 TEASPOON SEA SALT

1 TEASPOON FRESHLY GROUND BLACK PEPPER

2 GARLIC CLOVES, MINCED

8 OUNCES TURKEY TENDERLOIN

2 TABLESPOONS COCONUT OIL

1. Preheat the oven to 450°F.

2. In a small bowl, mix the rosemary, thyme, paprika, salt, pepper, and garlic. Rub the mixture evenly over the turkey.

3. Heat an ovenproof skillet over medium-high heat and add the coconut oil. Put the turkey in the pan and sear it on all sides until golden brown, about 7 minutes.

4. Transfer the skillet to the oven and roast the turkey for 15 minutes, or until the internal temperature of the turkey reaches 165°F. Let it rest for 5 minutes before slicing.

CALORIES: 247   TOTAL FAT: 16 G   SATURATED FAT: 12 G   SUGAR: 0 G   CARBOHYDRATES: 2 G

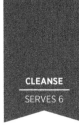

Lamb Vindaloo

Vindaloo is a classic curry dish from India. It may be a bit spicy, so leave out the cayenne pepper if you prefer milder food.

1 TABLESPOON COCONUT OIL

4 ONIONS, THINLY SLICED

4 GARLIC CLOVES, MINCED

¼ CUP FRESHLY SQUEEZED
    LEMON JUICE

2 TABLESPOONS WHOLE CUMIN SEEDS

½ TEASPOON CAYENNE PEPPER

1 TEASPOON DRY MUSTARD POWDER

½ TEASPOON TURMERIC

SEA SALT

½ CUP WATER

2 POUNDS BONELESS LAMB, CUT INTO
    BITE-SIZE PIECES

1. In a large pot, heat the coconut oil over medium heat. Add the onions and garlic, and sauté them until they are soft and slightly browned, 8 to 10 minutes.

2. In a small bowl, mix the lemon juice, cumin, cayenne, mustard powder, turmeric, and salt. Add the spice mixture, water, and lamb to the pot with the onions.

3. Reduce the heat to low, cover, and simmer the mixture for 1 hour, checking it occasionally to make sure the cooking liquid doesn't evaporate entirely. Add more water if necessary. Serve hot.

CALORIES: 257   TOTAL FAT: 11 G   SATURATED FAT: 5 G   SUGAR: 0 G   CARBOHYDRATES: 8 G

Slow-Roasted Lamb Shoulder with Lemons

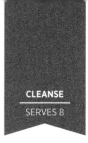

Cooking the lamb shoulder for a few hours turns the meat incredibly tender. This is the perfect dish to make for a Sunday supper, so you'll have leftovers for the next few days.

4 LEMONS

3 TABLESPOONS OLIVE OIL

1 (2- TO 2½-POUND) BONELESS
    LAMB SHOULDER, TIED WITH
    COOKING TWINE

½ TEASPOON SEA SALT

¼ TEASPOON FRESHLY GROUND
    BLACK PEPPER

4 CUPS LOW-SODIUM GLUTEN-FREE
    CHICKEN BROTH

1. Preheat the oven to 350°F.

2. Line a baking sheet with parchment paper.

3. Grate 1 teaspoon of lemon zest and set aside. Cut the lemons in half and toss them with 1 tablespoon of olive oil. Place the lemon halves on the lined baking sheet and set aside. Season the lamb with salt and pepper.

4. In a Dutch oven set over medium-high heat, heat the remaining 2 tablespoons of olive oil until hot. Add the lamb and brown it on all sides, about 10 minutes.

5. Add the broth and lemon zest and bring the mixture to a boil. Cover and transfer the Dutch oven to the oven.

6. Roast the lamb for about 2 hours, or until the lamb is tender, turning the meat several times.

7. After 1 hour, place the pan with the lemons on the bottom rack of the oven. When the lamb is done, the lemons should be browned and juicy.

8. Transfer the lamb to a serving platter and set the Dutch oven on the stovetop. Bring the liquid to a boil over high heat. Cook until it is reduced to about 2 cups.

9. Serve the lamb with the reduced liquid and roasted lemons.

CALORIES: 211   TOTAL FAT: 12 G   SATURATED FAT: 4 G   SUGAR: 0 G   CARBOHYDRATES: 5 G

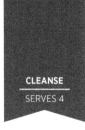

Grilled Beef Skewers with Zucchini

Sirloin is a less expensive cut of beef that is nice and lean. This whole dinner cooks in a single grill pan or outside on a grill.

8 OUNCES SIRLOIN STEAK, CUT INTO
    1½-INCH CUBES
2 ZUCCHINI, HALVED AND CUT
    INTO SPEARS
SEA SALT
FRESHLY GROUND BLACK PEPPER

EXTRA-VIRGIN OLIVE OIL
½ CUP FRESH MINT LEAVES, CUT
    INTO RIBBONS
½ TEASPOON RED CHILI FLAKES
1 LIME, CUT INTO WEDGES

1. Preheat a grill pan or the grill to medium-high heat.

2. Thread the beef and zucchini spears onto skewers.

3. Season the beef and zucchini spears with salt and pepper and drizzle them with oil.

4. Grill the beef and zucchini, turning regularly, until cooked through, 6 to 8 minutes.

5. Top the beef and zucchini with mint leaves and chili flakes. Serve with lime wedges on the side.

CALORIES: 159   TOTAL FAT: 8 G   SATURATED FAT: 3 G   SUGAR: 2 G   CARBOHYDRATES: 4 G

Grilled Sirloin with Garlic Butter

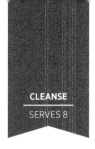

The classic way steak is served at a fancy restaurant is simply prepared with a pat of butter on top. The addition of garlic to this preparation adds even more flavor.

4 TABLESPOONS BUTTER

2 TEASPOONS GARLIC POWDER

4 GARLIC CLOVES, MINCED

3 POUNDS BEEF TOP SIRLOIN STEAKS

SEA SALT

FRESHLY GROUND BLACK PEPPER

1. Heat your outdoor grill to high heat, or preheat the broiler.

2. In a small saucepan over medium-low heat, melt the butter and add the garlic powder and garlic. Set aside.

3. Season the steak with salt and pepper. Grill or broil the steak for 4 to 5 minutes per side, or until it reaches your desired doneness.

4. Transfer the steak to a plate and brush the top with the garlic butter. Let it rest for 5 minutes before serving.

CALORIES: 513   TOTAL FAT: 24 G   SATURATED FAT: 11 G   SUGAR: 0 G   CARBOHYDRATES: 1 G

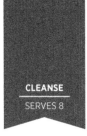

Lemony Pot Roast

Chuck roast is the cut of meat most often used for pot roasts. Find beef from a cow that was grass-fed and you'll realize how much more flavor it has.

2½ POUNDS CHUCK ROAST

1½ CUPS WATER

½ CUP FRESHLY SQUEEZED
   LEMON JUICE

1 ONION, CHOPPED

1 TEASPOON SEA SALT

1 TEASPOON CELERY SEEDS

1 TEASPOON ONION POWDER

¼ TEASPOON FRESHLY GROUND
   BLACK PEPPER

¼ TEASPOON DRIED MARJORAM

2 GARLIC CLOVES, CRUSHED

3 SLICES FRESH LEMON

1. Put the roast in a shallow pan.

2. In a medium bowl, combine the water, lemon juice, onion, salt, celery seed, onion powder, pepper, marjoram, garlic, and lemon slices. Pour the mixture over the meat, cover, and allow it to marinate in the refrigerator for 4 hours (or up to 24 hours).

3. Preheat the oven to 325°F.

4. Remove the roast from the marinade. Put it in a roasting pan and cover it with foil. Discard the marinade.

5. Roast the chuck roast for 1½ to 2 hours, or until it is tender when pierced with a fork. Let it rest for 15 minutes before slicing.

CALORIES: 430   TOTAL FAT: 28 G   SATURATED FAT: 2 G   SUGAR: 0 G   CARBOHYDRATES: 3 G

Sweet Potato Colcannon

If you do not like the taste of kale, this recipe can also be made with shredded cabbage. You will have to cook the cabbage longer than the kale to get a tender-crisp texture, so allot a bit more preparation time. The best cabbage to use for colcannon is green or savoy instead of red, which would create a strange color when mixed with the sweet potato.

6 SWEET POTATOES (ABOUT
    2 POUNDS), PEELED AND CUT
    INTO CHUNKS
¼ CUP BUTTER
1 BUNCH KALE, FINELY CHOPPED
    (ABOUT 5 CUPS)

4 GREEN ONIONS, FINELY CHOPPED
SEA SALT
FRESHLY GROUND BLACK PEPPER
2 TABLESPOONS CHOPPED
    FRESH PARSLEY

1. Place the sweet potatoes in a large pot of water over high heat. Bring the water to a boil, then reduce the heat and simmer the potatoes until they are fork tender, about 15 minutes.

2. While the potatoes are boiling, place a large skillet over medium-high heat and melt the butter.

3. Sauté the kale and green onions until they wilt and soften, about 3 minutes.

4. Drain the sweet potatoes and mash them until they are still a little chunky.

5. Add the kale mixture, including any liquid in the skillet, and stir to combine well.

6. Season the mixture with salt and pepper.

7. Serve the sweet potatoes topped with fresh parsley.

CALORIES: 383   TOTAL FAT: 12 G   SATURATED FAT: 7 G   SUGAR: 2 G   CARBOHYDRATES: 66 G

Spicy Vegetarian Chili

Chili is a staple comfort food in many households because it is incredibly simple to make and keeps very well in the fridge for days. If you want a satisfying meal waiting for you after a busy day, you can make this recipe in a slow cooker. Just combine all the ingredients in the slow cooker and cook on low or high depending on your schedule.

1 SWEET ONION, PEELED AND DICED

1 TEASPOON OLIVE OIL

1 TABLESPOON MINCED GARLIC

4 LARGE TOMATOES, DICED

1 (16-OUNCE) CAN SODIUM-FREE BLACK BEANS, DRAINED AND RINSED

1 (16-OUNCE) CAN SODIUM-FREE PINTO BEANS, DRAINED AND RINSED

1 (16-OUNCE) CAN SODIUM-FREE KIDNEY BEANS, DRAINED AND RINSED

1 (16-OUNCE) CAN SODIUM-FREE CHICKPEAS, DRAINED AND RINSED

3 TABLESPOONS CHILI SEASONING

1 TEASPOON GROUND CUMIN

PINCH CAYENNE

1. In a large pot over medium-high heat, sauté the onion in the olive oil until it softens, about 3 minutes.

2. Add the garlic and sauté an additional 2 minutes.

3. Stir in the tomatoes, black beans, pinto beans, kidney beans, chickpeas, chili seasoning, cumin, and cayenne, and bring the chili to a boil.

4. Simmer until the flavors mellow, stirring occasionally, about 45 minutes to 1 hour.

5. Remove the chili from the heat and let it sit for about 15 minutes before serving.

CALORIES: 316   TOTAL FAT: 3 G   SATURATED FAT: 0 G   SUGAR: 8 G   CARBOHYDRATES: 58 G

Curried Quinoa

Quinoa is a nutrition superstar that can be a staple ingredient in many of your dishes. It is high in protein and also a complex carbohydrate low on the glycemic index. Quinoa can be an expensive ingredient, so if you see a good deal, stock up and store it in a sealed container in your freezer for up to six months.

3 TABLESPOONS BUTTER

1 SWEET ONION, PEELED AND
    FINELY DICED

2 TEASPOONS MINCED GARLIC

1 TEASPOON GRATED FRESH GINGER

1 CUP DRY QUINOA, RINSED

2 CUPS LOW-SODIUM
    VEGETABLE BROTH

1 TABLESPOON CURRY POWDER

1 TEASPOON GROUND CUMIN

½ TEASPOON GROUND CORIANDER

1 CUP CHOPPED BROCCOLI

1 CUP PEAS, CANNED OR FROZEN

1 CUP SHREDDED SPINACH

1. In a large saucepan over medium-high heat, melt 2 tablespoons of butter and sauté the onion, garlic, and ginger until they are softened, about 3 minutes.

2. Add the quinoa and stir to mix.

3. Add the vegetable broth, curry powder, cumin, and coriander, and bring the liquid to a boil.

4. Reduce the heat to low and cover the pot. Simmer the quinoa until most of the liquid is absorbed, about 15 minutes.

5. While the quinoa is cooking, melt the remaining 1 tablespoon of butter in a skillet over medium heat, and sauté the broccoli, peas, and spinach until they are softened, about 3 minutes.

6. Add the cooked quinoa to the vegetables in the skillet and stir to mix well. Serve immediately.

CALORIES: 263   TOTAL FAT: 12 G   SATURATED FAT: 6 G   SUGAR: 2 G   CARBOHYDRATES: 34 G

Roasted Chicken with Pears

When you're ready to eat some fruit again, don't forget to use it in savory dishes. The pears bring a wonderful sweetness to a classic roasted chicken.

1 WHOLE CHICKEN (ABOUT 3½ POUNDS), RINSED AND PATTED DRY (DISCARD NECK, LIVER, AND GIBLETS)
SEA SALT
FRESHLY GROUND BLACK PEPPER
1 TABLESPOON FRESH THYME LEAVES, PLUS 10 SPRIGS FRESH THYME
3 GARLIC CLOVES, UNPEELED
½ LEMON, HALVED
8 SHALLOTS, PEELED AND HALVED LENGTHWISE
3 ANJOU PEARS, CORED AND QUARTERED

1. Preheat the oven to 475°F.

2. Put the chicken in a roasting pan and season it with salt and pepper. Gently loosen the skin over the breasts and rub the thyme leaves, salt, and pepper under the skin.

3. Stuff the cavity with 5 thyme sprigs, garlic, and lemon. Use kitchen twine to tie the legs together and tuck the wing tips underneath.

4. Roast the chicken for 15 minutes.

5. Remove it from the oven and baste it with the pan juice. Add the shallots, pears, and remaining thyme sprigs to the pan.

6. Put the pan back in oven and roast the chicken for 30 minutes. Baste the bird and remove the pears and shallots. Set aside.

7. Return the chicken to the oven for another 15 to 30 minutes, or until the thick part of the thigh registers 165°F on a meat thermometer.

8. Let the chicken rest for 10 minutes before cutting it. Serve the chicken with the roasted pears and shallots on the side.

CALORIES: 181   TOTAL FAT: 3 G   SATURATED FAT: 1 G   SUGAR: 0 G   CARBOHYDRATES: 23 G

Herbed Chicken with White Beans

When cooking with canned beans, don't forget to rinse them well. They come packed in a salty liquid, and rinsing helps get rid of a lot of the extra sodium.

FOR THE MARINADE

⅓ CUP OLIVE OIL

3 GARLIC CLOVES, MINCED

2 TABLESPOONS FRESHLY SQUEEZED
    LEMON JUICE

4 SPRIGS FRESH OREGANO

4 SPRIGS FRESH TARRAGON

4 SPRIGS FRESH BASIL

4 SPRIGS FRESH PARSLEY

2 SPRIGS FRESH ROSEMARY

FRESHLY GROUND BLACK PEPPER

FOR THE CHICKEN

2 POUNDS BONELESS, SKINLESS
    CHICKEN BREASTS, CUT INTO
    1-INCH CUBES

2 TABLESPOONS OLIVE OIL

½ RED ONION, THINLY SLICED

1½ CUPS CANNED SODIUM-FREE
    WHITE CANNELLINI BEANS,
    DRAINED AND RINSED

SEA SALT

FRESHLY GROUND BLACK PEPPER

To make the marinade:

1. In a food processor, add the olive oil, garlic, lemon juice, and the leaves from the oregano, tarragon, basil, parsley, and rosemary. Season with the pepper.

2. Blend the mixture until it becomes a smooth green paste. If the mixture looks too thick, add a few spoonfuls of water.

To make the chicken:

1. Pour the marinade over the chicken and refrigerate it, covered, for at least 2 hours or overnight.

2. Heat 2 tablespoons of olive oil in a large pan over moderate heat. When the oil is hot, add the cubed chicken and brown it lightly, about 3 minutes. Discard any remaining marinade.

3. Add the onion and sauté it for 2 minutes, or until the onion begins to soften. Add the beans and cook the mixture for 2 minutes more, or until the chicken is cooked through. Season the chicken and beans with salt and pepper.

CALORIES: 370   TOTAL FAT: 18 G   SATURATED FAT: 3 G   SUGAR: 1 G   CARBOHYDRATES: 12 G

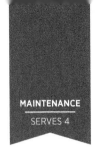

Broiled Lemon Chicken

Lemon is one of the most popular flavors in the world for both savory and sweet dishes. The bright citrus taste of this marinade is perfect for chicken, especially when combined with fresh thyme. Lemon is an effective detoxifier and boosts the immune system, which is very important when fighting candida.

½ CUP FRESHLY SQUEEZED
    LEMON JUICE

¼ CUP OLIVE OIL

2 TABLESPOONS CHOPPED
    FRESH THYME

½ TEASPOON SEA SALT

½ TEASPOON FRESHLY GROUND
    BLACK PEPPER

2 DROPS LIQUID STEVIA

1 POUND BONELESS SKINLESS
    CHICKEN BREASTS, HALVED

1. In a medium bowl, whisk together the lemon juice, olive oil, thyme, sea salt, pepper, and stevia until they are well blended.

2. Place the chicken in a large sealable freezer bag and pour in the marinade.

3. Squeeze the excess air out of the bag and place it in the fridge for at least 4 hours to marinate.

4. Preheat oven to 400°F.

5. Place the chicken in a 9-by-13-inch baking dish, shaking off the excess marinade. Discard the marinade.

6. Bake the chicken until it is cooked through, 20 to 25 minutes. Serve immediately with your choice of vegetables.

CALORIES: 335   TOTAL FAT: 21 G   SATURATED FAT: 4 G   SUGAR: 1 G   CARBOHYDRATES: 2 G

Savory Stuffed Tomatoes with Turkey

Vegetables, such as tomatoes, make convenient, appealing containers for any filling. You just need to make sure you don't overcook the vegetables, or the entire dish can collapse. If you prefer a vegetarian option, you can substitute brown rice for the turkey. Use about two cups of rice and increase the amount of carrots to create some moisture and bulk.

8 FIRM TOMATOES

1 POUND EXTRA-LEAN
    GROUND TURKEY

1 SWEET ONION, PEELED AND
    FINELY DICED

1 CELERY STALK, FINELY DICED

1 TEASPOON MINCED GARLIC

½ CUP COARSELY SHREDDED CARROT

½ CUP SHREDDED SPINACH

2 TEASPOONS CHOPPED
    FRESH CILANTRO

½ TEASPOON GROUND CUMIN

½ TEASPOON FRESHLY GROUND
    BLACK PEPPER

¼ TEASPOON SEA SALT

1. Preheat the oven to 350°F.

2. Cut the tops off the tomatoes and carefully scoop out the insides without breaking the tomato skin.

3. Reserve half the tomato insides for the filling and place the rest in a sealed container for another recipe. Chop the reserved tomato insides coarsely and set aside.

4. Turn the tomatoes upside down onto paper towels and let them drain for about 30 minutes.

5. Place a large skillet over medium-high heat and brown the turkey until it is completely cooked through, 6 to 7 minutes.

6. Add the onion, celery, and garlic to the turkey in the skillet and sauté until the vegetables are softened, about 3 minutes.

continued ▶

7. Add the reserved tomato, carrot, spinach, cilantro, cumin, pepper, and salt and cook until the spinach is wilted, about 3 minutes. Remove the skillet from the heat.

8. Place the tomatoes hollow-side up in a baking dish and evenly divide the turkey filling among the tomatoes.

9. Bake the stuffed tomatoes for about 45 minutes or until the tomatoes are soft.

10. Serve 2 tomatoes per person with a tossed salad or brown rice.

CALORIES: 187   TOTAL FAT: 3 G   SATURATED FAT: 1 G   SUGAR: 8 G   CARBOHYDRATES: 13 G

Turkey Cabbage Rolls

Stuffed cabbage rolls are a classic comfort food, and this version is packed with protein and vitamins. This dish takes a little longer to prepare, since you have to make the sauce ahead of time, but make a big batch of sauce and freeze half so you can cut out that step the next time.

FOR THE MARINARA SAUCE

2 TEASPOONS OLIVE OIL

3 CUPS CHOPPED ONIONS

¾ CUP DICED CARROT

½ CUP DICED CELERY

¼ CUP MINCED GARLIC

3 TABLESPOONS CHOPPED
    FRESH OREGANO

2 TABLESPOONS NO-SALT, NO-SUGAR-
    ADDED TOMATO PASTE

5½ POUNDS PLUM TOMATOES, PEELED
    AND CHOPPED

¾ CUP CHOPPED FRESH BASIL

1½ TEASPOONS SEA SALT

½ TEASPOON FRESHLY GROUND
    BLACK PEPPER

FOR THE CABBAGE ROLLS

1 YELLOW ONION, SLICED

1 EGGPLANT, CUT INTO CUBES

1 ZUCCHINI, CUT INTO CUBES

1 RED BELL PEPPER, SEEDED
    AND CHOPPED

1 YELLOW BELL PEPPER, SEEDED
    AND CHOPPED

2 CARROTS, PEELED AND CHOPPED

1 PARSNIP, PEELED AND CHOPPED

2 GARLIC CLOVES, MINCED

2 TEASPOONS OLIVE OIL

½ TEASPOON DRIED THYME

¼ TEASPOON DRIED BASIL

¼ TEASPOON DRIED OREGANO

1 HEAD GREEN CABBAGE

1 POUND FRESHLY GROUND TURKEY

To make the marinara sauce:

1. Place a large skillet over medium-high heat. Add the oil and swirl to coat the skillet.

2. Add the onion, carrot, celery, garlic, and oregano, and sauté for 8 minutes.

3. Add the tomato paste and cook for 2 minutes, stirring frequently.

4. Add the plum tomatoes, lower the heat, cover, and cook for 30 minutes.

continued ▶

5. Use an immersion blender (or transfer the mixture to a blender) and purée the tomatoes until they are a smooth consistency.

6. Add the basil, salt, and pepper and cook uncovered on high for another 30 minutes. Remove the sauce from the heat and set aside.

To make the cabbage rolls:

1. Preheat the oven to 425°F.

2. On a large baking sheet, combine the onion, eggplant, zucchini, bell peppers, carrots, parsnip, garlic, olive oil, thyme, basil, and oregano. Toss until the vegetables are evenly coated.

3. Roast the vegetables for 30 minutes, stirring halfway through.

4. While the vegetables are roasting, remove the core from the cabbage. Fill a large pot with water and bring it to a boil. Put the cabbage in the water, cover, and boil it for 6 to 7 minutes.

5. Drain the cabbage in a colander and remove the large outer leaves. Cut out the thick stems from the large leaves.

6. In a large sauté pan set over medium heat, brown the turkey, stirring regularly until it is cooked through. Add 1 cup of marinara sauce and all the roasted vegetables. Stir to combine.

7. Reduce the oven temperature to 375°F.

8. Pour 1 cup of marinara evenly over the bottom of a shallow baking dish.

9. Taking 1 cabbage leaf at a time, spoon ½ cup of the turkey-vegetable filling onto one end of the leaf, roll it up, and place it seam-side down in the baking dish. Repeat with the remaining leaves and filling.

10. Pour 1 cup of marinara sauce over the cabbage rolls and bake them uncovered for 40 minutes. Let the rolls rest for 5 minutes before serving.

CALORIES: 272   TOTAL FAT: 8 G   SATURATED FAT: 2 G   SUGAR: 4 G   CARBOHYDRATES: 39 G

Chili Turkey Burgers

If you want a more classic burger, you can source out candida diet–friendly buns or make your own instead of serving these patties on lettuce. The jalapeño pepper in the burgers creates a lovely heat and adds complexity to the dish that can be enhanced if you use a barbeque instead of the oven.

1 POUND GROUND LEAN
   TURKEY BREAST
1 CARROT, SHREDDED AND THE LIQUID
   SQUEEZED OUT
½ RED ONION, PEELED AND
   FINELY DICED
½ JALAPEÑO PEPPER, MINCED
1 TABLESPOON CHOPPED FRESH
   CILANTRO

1 TEASPOON CHILI POWDER
1 TEASPOONS CUMIN
¼ TEASPOON FRESHLY GROUND
   BLACK PEPPER
¼ TEASPOON SEA SALT
LETTUCE, FOR SERVING
CHOPPED TOMATO, FOR SERVING
SLICED RED ONION, FOR SERVING

1. Preheat oven to 400°F.

2. Line a baking sheet with foil. Set aside.

3. In a large bowl, combine the turkey, carrot, onion, jalapeño, and cilantro. Add in the chili powder, cumin, pepper, and salt, and stir until they are well combined.

4. Form the turkey mixture into 4 patties and place them on the baking sheet.

5. Bake the patties in the oven, turning once, until the burgers are cooked through but still juicy, about 20 minutes.

6. Serve the burgers on lettuce leaves with chopped tomato and sliced red onion.

CALORIES: 156   TOTAL FAT: 3 G   SATURATED FAT: 1 G   SUGAR: 1 G   CARBOHYDRATES: 3 G

Traditional Meatloaf

For a variation on this traditional dish, you can substitute lean ground chicken or turkey for the beef in this recipe. You might want to make an extra meatloaf to have on hand the next day for a cold sandwich on approved bread. This recipe also freezes beautifully if you cool the meatloaf completely before storing it in a sealed plastic bag.

NONSTICK COOKING SPRAY

1 POUND EXTRA-LEAN GROUND BEEF

2 EGGS

1 SWEET ONION, PEELED AND
    FINELY DICED

1 CARROT, PEELED AND SHREDDED

⅓ CUP OAT BRAN

2 TEASPOONS MINCED GARLIC

2 TEASPOONS CHOPPED FRESH THYME

½ TEASPOON SEA SALT

¼ TEASPOON FRESHLY GROUND
    BLACK PEPPER

1. Preheat oven to 350°F.

2. Spray a 9-by-5-inch loaf pan with nonstick cooking spray and set aside.

3. In a medium bowl, combine the beef, eggs, onion, carrot, oat bran, garlic, thyme, salt, and pepper until well mixed.

4. Press the meat mixture into the loaf pan and bake it until the meatloaf is cooked through, about 1 hour.

5. Remove the meatloaf from the oven and let it sit for about 10 minutes, then pour off any extra oil in the pan. Slice the meatloaf and serve.

CALORIES: 296   TOTAL FAT: 11 G   SATURATED FAT: 4 G   SUGAR: 3 G   CARBOHYDRATES: 12 G

NOTES

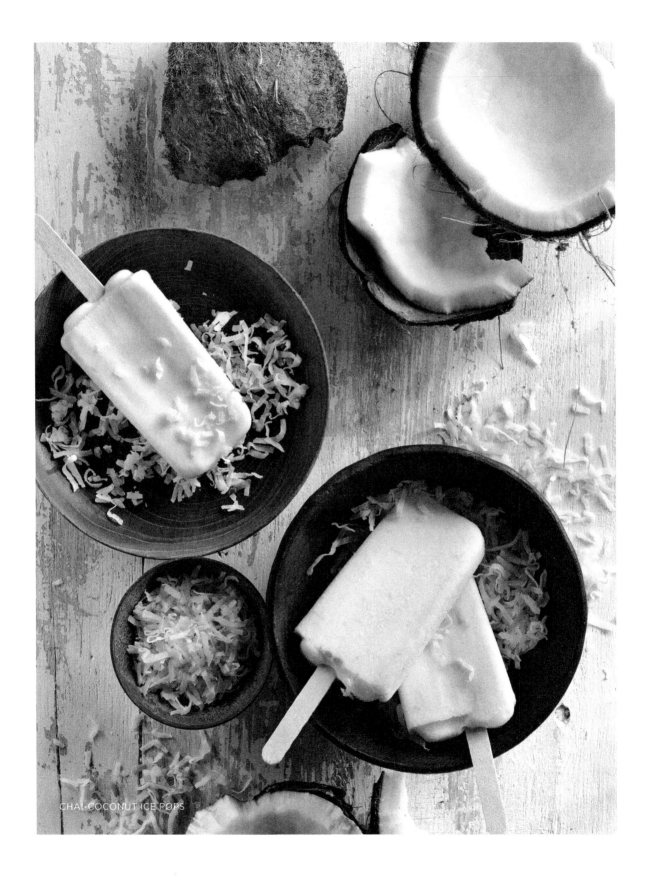

CHAI-COCONUT ICE POPS

10

Desserts

CLEANSE

FRESH MINT BARS

CHAI-COCONUT ICE POPS

I SCREAM FOR VANILLA ICE CREAM

CHOCOLATE "MILKSHAKE"

NUTTY COCONUT BARK

MAINTENANCE

CHIA SEED AND COCONUT PUDDING WITH STRAWBERRIES

STRAWBERRY SHORTCAKE

WARM APPLE BAKE WITH STREUSEL TOPPING

ALMOND-CHOCOLATE TRUFFLES

MIXED-BERRY SLUSHIE

Fresh Mint Bars

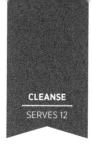

Mint and chocolate are two flavors that go together perfectly. This three-layer bar mimics the flavor of your favorite candies and cookies without any bad-for-you ingredients. The best way to include stevia in dishes is to add a little, taste it, and add a little more if you need it. Too much and the final dish will taste bitter.

FOR THE BOTTOM LAYER

¾ CUP RAW SUNFLOWER SEEDS

¼ CUP SHREDDED UNSWEETENED
    COCONUT

2 TABLESPOONS COCONUT BUTTER

1 TEASPOON SUNFLOWER SEED
    BUTTER

DASH SEA SALT

FOR THE MIDDLE LAYER

1½ AVOCADOS, PEELED AND PITTED

6 FRESH MINT LEAVES

2 CUPS SPINACH LEAVES

½ TEASPOON MINT EXTRACT

¼ CUP COCONUT BUTTER

DASH LIQUID STEVIA

FOR THE TOP LAYER

3 TABLESPOONS COCONUT OIL

3 TABLESPOONS COCONUT BUTTER

¼ CUP UNSWEETENED FULL-FAT
    COCONUT MILK

½ TEASPOON MINT EXTRACT

DASH LIQUID STEVIA

To make the bottom layer:

1. In a food processor, grind the sunflower seeds.

2. Add the coconut, coconut butter, sunflower seed butter, and salt and blend until the mixture is crumbly and combined.

3. Spread the mixture in the bottom of a silicone loaf pan and put in the freezer to firm up.

To make the middle layer:

1. Combine the avocado, mint, spinach, mint extract, coconut butter, and stevia in a food processor and blend until smooth.

2. Spread the mixture over the bottom layer and return the pan to the freezer. Clean the food processor before proceeding to the next step.

continued ▶

To make the top layer:

1. Soften the coconut oil and coconut butter in a saucepan over medium-low heat.

2. Pour the coconut mixture into the food processor and add the coconut milk, mint extract, and stevia. Blend until it is thick and smooth.

3. Spread the mixture over the middle layer and put the loaf pan back in the freezer to firm up.

To make the bars:

1. When all 3 layers are frozen through, cut the loaf into 12 bars.

2. Store the bars in an airtight container in the refrigerator for up to 3 days.

CALORIES: 241   TOTAL FAT: 23 G   SATURATED FAT: 15 G   SUGAR: 2 G   CARBOHYDRATES: 9 G

Chai-Coconut Ice Pops

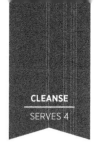

You'll need ice pop molds to make this recipe. You can find them in kitchen supply stores and department stores, and they come in lots of fun shapes.

1½ CUPS CANNED UNSWEETENED
    COCONUT MILK

DASH LIQUID STEVIA

½ TEASPOON GROUND CARDAMOM

1 TEASPOON CINNAMON

¼ TEASPOON GROUND NUTMEG

1 TEASPOON ALCOHOL-FREE
    VANILLA EXTRACT

1. In a medium bowl, whisk together all the ingredients until they are blended.

2. Pour it evenly into 4 ice pop molds and freeze until they are solid.

CALORIES: 96   TOTAL FAT: 9 G   SATURATED FAT: 9 G   SUGAR: 0 G   CARBOHYDRATES: 1 G

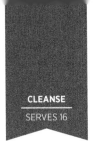

I Scream for Vanilla Ice Cream

Like most ice creams, this dessert is higher in fat and calories than some other dessert choices. Enjoy it in moderation to satisfy your frozen dessert craving.

1½ CUPS COCONUT OIL

1½ STICKS UNSALTED BUTTER

12 EGGS

1 TABLESPOON ALCOHOL-FREE VANILLA EXTRACT

½ TEASPOON POWDERED STEVIA

1. In a saucepan over medium heat, melt the coconut oil and butter, stirring until they are combined. Set aside until cool.

2. In a blender, combine the eggs, vanilla, stevia, and coconut oil and butter mixture. Blend until smooth.

3. Pour the mixture into a 9-by-13-inch glass pan with a lid, and freeze it for 6 hours.

4. Remove the glass pan from the freezer and score the top of the ice cream with a knife to mark out 16 squares.

5. To serve, let the ice cream thaw on the counter for 10 to 15 minutes, then remove 1 of the servings.

CALORIES: 312   TOTAL FAT: 33 G   SATURATED FAT: 25 G   SUGAR: 1 G   CARBOHYDRATES: 1 G

Chocolate "Milkshake"

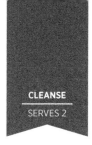

Don't worry about the avocado in this dessert; the flavor disappears and it makes the final dish creamy and indulgent.

2½ CUPS UNSWEETENED
    ALMOND MILK

1 RIPE AVOCADO, PEELED AND PITTED

2 TABLESPOONS UNSWEETENED
    COCOA POWDER

1 TEASPOON CINNAMON

1 TEASPOON ALCOHOL-FREE
    VANILLA EXTRACT

LIQUID STEVIA

2 CUPS ICE CUBES

1. In a blender, combine the almond milk, avocado, cocoa powder, cinnamon, vanilla, and stevia. Blend until the mixture is smooth.

2. If you have a high-powered blender, add the ice and blend until smooth. Otherwise, pour the shake over the ice to drink.

CALORIES: 203   TOTAL FAT: 17 G   SATURATED FAT: 3 G   SUGAR: 1 G   CARBOHYDRATES: 13 G

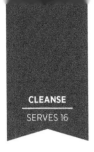
Nutty Coconut Bark

Coconut makes an appearance three times in this recipe—in coconut oil, coconut butter, and shredded coconut. We added almonds and pecans, but feel free to mix up the nuts based on your preference.

2 TABLESPOONS COCONUT OIL,
    PLUS 2 TEASPOONS
½ CUP SLIVERED ALMONDS
1 CUP WHOLE PECANS
PINCH SEA SALT
1½ CUPS COCONUT BUTTER

½ TEASPOON ALMOND EXTRACT
½ TEASPOON ALCOHOL-FREE
    VANILLA EXTRACT
1 CUP SHREDDED UNSWEETENED
    COCONUT

1. Line a 9-by-13-inch cookie pan with parchment paper.

2. In a cast-iron pan set over medium heat, melt 2 teaspoons of coconut oil. Add the almond slivers and pecans and reduce the heat to medium-low. Toast the nuts for 2 to 3 minutes, stirring frequently to prevent burning. Remove the nuts from the heat and sprinkle them with salt.

3. In the top of a double boiler set over simmering water, melt the coconut butter with the remaining 2 tablespoons of coconut oil. Add the almond extract, vanilla extract, and toasted nuts, and mix well.

4. Pour the mixture onto the prepared cookie pan, spreading evenly so it's in a thin layer. Press the shredded coconut on the top of the mixture and refrigerate it for 15 minutes. Remove the bark from the freezer and break it into pieces.

CALORIES: 261   TOTAL FAT: 26 G   SATURATED FAT: 18 G   SUGAR: 2 G   CARBOHYDRATES: 9 G

Chia Seed and Coconut Pudding with Strawberries

This dish is sweet and flavorful—perfect as a light dessert in summer when berries are in season. Make it earlier in the day, because it requires at least four hours to firm up.

½ CUP UNSWEETENED LIGHT
   COCONUT MILK
½ CUP UNSWEETENED ALMOND MILK
½ CUP SLICED FRESH STRAWBERRIES

1 TABLESPOON CHIA SEEDS
1 TABLESPOON SHREDDED
   UNSWEETENED COCONUT
2 DROPS LIQUID STEVIA

1. In a large bowl, combine all the ingredients and mix well.

2. Pour the mixture into a storage container, seal it, and put it in the refrigerator at least 4 hours or overnight.

CALORIES: 107   TOTAL FAT: 8 G   SATURATED FAT: 6 G   SUGAR: 4 G   CARBOHYDRATES: 8 G

Strawberry Shortcake

Who doesn't love this summer classic? For this dish, the standard shortcake biscuits get replaced with a coconut-and-almond-flour version that tastes great and satisfies your sweet tooth. Make sure your baking soda and baking powder are gluten-free, and always use alcohol-free vanilla extract.

1 TABLESPOON FRESHLY SQUEEZED LEMON JUICE

1 CUP UNSWEETENED COCONUT MILK

1½ TEASPOONS ALCOHOL-FREE VANILLA EXTRACT

3 TABLESPOONS FINELY GROUND FLAXSEED

12 DROPS LIQUID STEVIA

2 TABLESPOONS COCONUT OIL, PLUS MORE FOR BRUSHING, MELTED

½ CUP PLUS 2 TABLESPOONS COCONUT FLOUR

2 TABLESPOONS ALMOND FLOUR

PINCH SEA SALT

¾ TEASPOON BAKING POWDER

¾ TEASPOON BAKING SODA

16 STRAWBERRIES, SLICED

1. Preheat the oven to 400°F.

2. Line a baking sheet with parchment paper.

3. Pour the lemon juice into a measuring cup and fill up to the 1 cup mark with the coconut milk.

4. In a large bowl, combine the lemon and coconut milk with the vanilla, ground flax-seed, stevia, and melted coconut oil. Let the mixture sit for 3 minutes to thicken.

5. In a medium bowl, sift together the coconut flour, almond flour, salt, baking powder, and baking soda.

6. Pour the wet ingredients into the flour mixture and stir until just combined. Do not overmix—it's okay if the batter is a bit sticky.

7. Shape the dough into 8 flat, round biscuits. Place the biscuits on the prepared baking sheet and bake them for 12 minutes. Brush the tops with melted coconut oil and bake them for 12 to 15 minutes more, or until lightly browned. Serve the biscuits topped with sliced strawberries.

CALORIES: 171   TOTAL FAT: 11 G   SATURATED FAT: 6 G   SUGAR: 2 G   CARBOHYDRATES: 13 G

Warm Apple Bake with Streusel Topping

This dessert has everything you want on a chilly evening—sweet apples, spices, nuts, and butter. It looks complicated but comes together easily.

FOR THE CRUST

1¾ CUPS ALMOND FLOUR

1 TABLESPOON COCONUT FLOUR

¼ TEASPOON SEA SALT

6 TABLESPOONS BUTTER, AT ROOM
    TEMPERATURE

½ TEASPOON VANILLA

½ TEASPOON LIQUID STEVIA

FOR THE APPLE MIXTURE

8 CUPS PEELED AND CHOPPED APPLES

⅓ CUP CHOPPED WALNUTS

3 TEASPOONS CINNAMON

½ TEASPOON GROUND NUTMEG

¼ TEASPOON GROUND CLOVES

¼ TEASPOON GROUND GINGER

1 TABLESPOON COCONUT FLOUR

½ TEASPOON SEA SALT

8 TABLESPOONS BUTTER, AT ROOM
    TEMPERATURE

1 TEASPOON VANILLA

1 TEASPOON POWDERED STEVIA

FOR THE STREUSEL

½ CUP COCONUT FLOUR

½ CUP ALMOND FLOUR

¼ TEASPOON NUTMEG

½ TEASPOON CINNAMON

⅛ TEASPOON SEA SALT

½ TEASPOON POWDERED STEVIA

⅓ CUP CHOPPED ALMONDS

6 TABLESPOONS BUTTER, CUT
    INTO PIECES

1 TABLESPOON BEATEN EGG

To make the crust:

1. Preheat the oven to 350°F.

2. In a medium bowl, mix together the almond flour, coconut flour, salt, butter, vanilla, and stevia until it has a doughy consistency.

3. Spread the mixture evenly over the bottom of a 9-by-12-inch baking pan. Press the dough in with your fingers until it is even.

continued ▶

4. Bake the crust for 5 to 10 minutes, or until the edges are lightly browned. Remove the crust from the oven and set aside.

To make the apple mixture:

1. In a large bowl, mix the apples, walnuts, cinnamon, nutmeg, cloves, ginger, coconut flour, salt, butter, vanilla, and stevia until the apple pieces are evenly coated.

2. Set aside while you make the streusel.

To make the streusel:

1. In a medium bowl, combine the coconut flour, almond flour, nutmeg, cinnamon, salt, stevia, almonds, butter, and egg.

2. Mix the ingredients with your hands until the mixture forms large crumbs.

To put it all together:

1. Pour the apple mixture into the prebaked crust, then sprinkle the streusel mixture evenly over the top.

2. Cover the streusel with foil and bake it at 350°F for 30 minutes, or until the apples are softened. Uncover and bake the streusel for 10 to 15 more minutes, or until the top is toasted.

3. Let it sit for 10 minutes before serving, so the apples can set.

CALORIES: 324   TOTAL FAT: 27 G   SATURATED FAT: 10 G   SUGAR: 7 G   CARBOHYDRATES: 18 G

Almond-Chocolate Truffles

Cauliflower in a dessert? The vegetable is actually the secret to the perfect texture in these truffles. Store them in the freezer. Just microwave your truffle for twelve seconds whenever a craving hits and it will be perfect to eat.

FOR THE TRUFFLES
½ HEAD CAULIFLOWER
2 TABLESPOONS NO-SUGAR-ADDED
    ALMOND BUTTER
½ CUP SHREDDED UNSWEETENED
    COCONUT
2 TABLESPOONS UNSWEETENED
    CACAO NIBS
PINCH POWDERED STEVIA

FOR THE GLAZE
1 TABLESPOON COCONUT OIL
1 TABLESPOON NO-SUGAR-ADDED
    ALMOND BUTTER
2 TABLESPOONS COCOA POWDER
PINCH STEVIA

To make the truffles:

1. Chop the cauliflower into small pieces and pulse it in a food processor until it resembles rice. Add the almond butter, coconut, cacao nibs, and stevia to the cauliflower and pulse to mix.

2. Shape the dough into 8 balls and freeze them on a cookie sheet.

To make the glaze:

1. Melt the coconut oil in a small saucepan over medium heat. Whisk in the almond butter, cacao powder, and stevia.

2. Dip the frozen truffles in the glaze and set them on a cookie sheet lined with wax paper. Freeze the truffles until they are firm.

CALORIES: 277   TOTAL FAT: 21 G   SATURATED FAT: 14 G   SUGAR: 2 G   CARBOHYDRATES: 18 G

Mixed-Berry Slushie

When you're ready to enjoy berries again, feature them in this refreshing dessert. The best part: You can always have the ingredients on hand, since the dish uses frozen fruit.

2 CUPS FROZEN BLUEBERRIES

2 CUPS FROZEN RASPBERRIES

½ CUP FROZEN CRANBERRIES

1½ CUPS WATER

10 DROPS STEVIA

½ TEASPOON ALCOHOL-FREE
    VANILLA EXTRACT

1. Put all the ingredients in a high-powered blender and purée until smooth. Stop and push the mixture down the sides with a spoon several times when blending.

2. Serve immediately.

CALORIES: 77   TOTAL FAT: 1 G   SATURATED FAT: 0 G   SUGAR: 7 G   CARBOHYDRATES: 18 G

NOTES

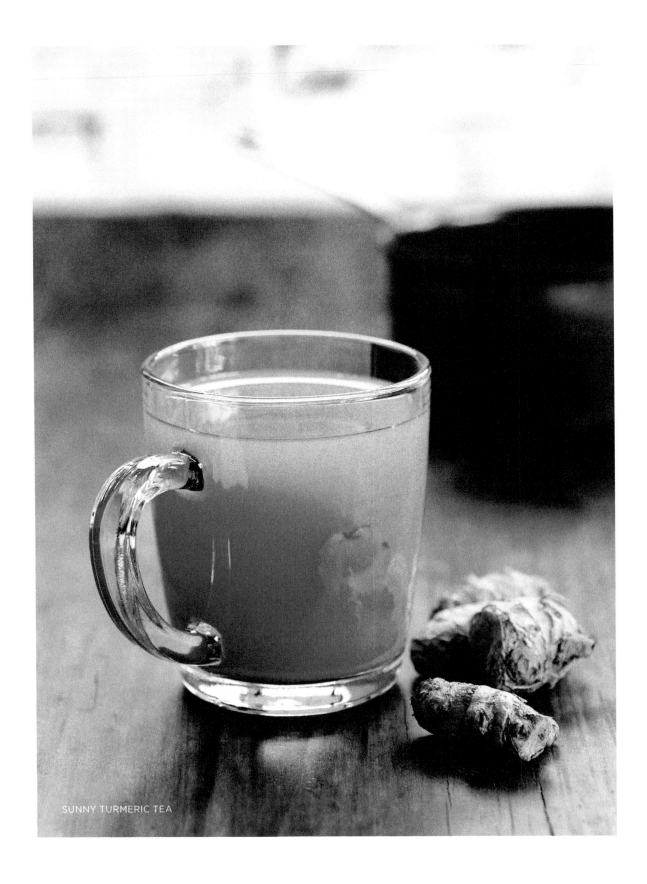
SUNNY TURMERIC TEA

11

Beverages

CLEANSE

SIMPLE GINGER TEA

SUNNY TURMERIC TEA

AVOCADO-COCONUT SMOOTHIE

SAVORY GREEN HERB JUICE

CREAMY COCONUT MILK

MAINTENANCE

CHAI LATTE

REFRESHING LEMON-LIMEADE

ICY VANILLA MILKSHAKE

SIMPLE CITRUS-SPINACH COCKTAIL

Simple Ginger Tea

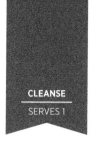

Ginger should be consumed every day when you are on a candida diet because it can be very effective for soothing the digestive inflammation associated with this condition. Ginger is also a proven detoxifier, and this tea can be perfect to kick-start your day or wind down at night. Ginger tea can be served cold over ice with fresh mint or a slice of lemon.

2 CUPS WATER

1 (1-INCH) PIECE FRESH GINGER ROOT,
    PEELED AND FINELY GRATED

¼ FRESH LEMON

1. Pour the water into a small saucepan over high heat and add the grated ginger.

2. Bring the water to a boil, then reduce the heat and simmer the ginger for about 30 minutes to infuse the water with the ginger.

3. Remove the pan from the heat and strain the tea through a fine sieve.

4. Squeeze the lemon into the tea and drink hot.

CALORIES: 10   TOTAL FAT: 0 G   SATURATED FAT: 0 G   SUGAR: 0 G   CARBOHYDRATES: 3 G

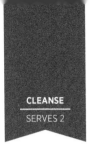

Sunny Turmeric Tea

Turmeric is found often in rice and grain dishes because it tints the other ingredients a glorious yellow color and has a pleasing taste. It is combined with other warm spices, such as cinnamon, ginger, cloves, cumin, and allspice, to create exotic blends. This tea should be consumed immediately after brewing because turmeric can get slightly bitter if it sits too long.

4 CUPS WATER

1½ TEASPOONS TURMERIC POWDER

¼ TEASPOON GROUND CINNAMON

¼ TEASPOON GROUND GINGER

PINCH GROUND CLOVE

PINCH STEVIA

1. Pour the water into a small saucepan and add the turmeric, cinnamon, ginger, clove, and stevia.

2. Bring the water to a boil over medium-high heat, then reduce the heat and simmer the tea for about 10 minutes to infuse the water.

3. Pour the tea through a fine sieve and serve hot.

CALORIES: 8   TOTAL FAT: 0 G   SATURATED FAT: 0 G   SUGAR: 0 G   CARBOHYDRATES: 3 G

Avocado-Coconut Smoothie

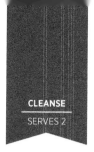

Smoothies can be satisfying meal replacements if you are time stressed or want a change from more traditional meals. The avocados in this recipe create a smooth milkshake-like texture and lovely pale green appearance. Make sure your avocados are ripe to ensure the correct consistency.

1 AVOCADO, PEELED AND PITTED

2 CUPS UNSWEETENED ALMOND MILK

PINCH GROUND CINNAMON

PINCH GROUND STEVIA

10 ICE CUBES

1. Place the avocado, almond milk, cinnamon, and stevia in a blender and pulse until smooth.

2. Add the ice to the blender and pulse until the smoothie is thick and smooth.

3. Pour the smoothie into 2 glasses and serve.

CALORIES: 235   TOTAL FAT: 22 G   SATURATED FAT: 4 G   SUGAR: 1 G   CARBOHYDRATES: 11 G

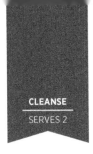
Savory Green Herb Juice

This vibrant green juice has a lovely fragrance that will remind you of a sun-warmed garden. Herbs have been used medicinally for centuries for many conditions as well as used to enhance the flavor of food. Thyme and garlic are both effective antifungals, which promote a healthy immune system and detoxify the body.

2 CELERY STALKS, CUT INTO CHUNKS

2 CUPS SPINACH

1 GARLIC CLOVE

2 SPRIGS FRESH BASIL

3 SPRIGS FRESH OREGANO

3 SPRIGS FRESH THYME

¼ CUP FRESHLY SQUEEZED
LEMON JUICE

2 CUPS WATER

1. Place the celery, spinach, garlic, basil, oregano, thyme leaves, lemon juice, and water in a blender and pulse until it is smooth.

2. Pour the juice into 2 glasses and serve.

CALORIES: 43   TOTAL FAT: 1 G   SATURATED FAT: 0 G   SUGAR: 1 G   CARBOHYDRATES: 8 G

Creamy Coconut Milk

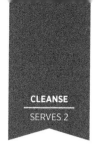

You may never purchase coconut milk again after seeing how simple it is to make at home. Once you master creating plain unsweetened coconut milk, you can experiment with vanilla beans, a couple drops of stevia, and spices, such as cinnamon and nutmeg.

3 CUPS VERY HOT
   (NOT BOILING) WATER

1½ CUPS SHREDDED
   UNSWEETENED COCONUT

1. Place the water and coconut in a blender and blend on low speed for about 2 minutes.

2. Increase the speed to high and blend an additional 3 minutes.

3. Strain the coconut milk through a fine sieve or cheesecloth.

4. Place the milk in the fridge until it is chilled before serving.

CALORIES: 142   TOTAL FAT: 13 G   SATURATED FAT: 12 G   SUGAR: 3 G   CARBOHYDRATES: 7 G

Chai Latte

This luscious drink does not actually contain any chai tea, but the combination of warm spices will make you think you are enjoying a sugary treat from a high-end coffee shop. If you like your latte sweeter, adjust the stevia proportions before adding the ice.

3 CUPS UNSWEETENED ALMOND MILK

1 AVOCADO, PEELED, PITTED, AND HALVED

20 DROPS LIQUID STEVIA

1 TEASPOON ALCOHOL-FREE VANILLA EXTRACT

1 TEASPOON GROUND CINNAMON

½ TEASPOON GROUND NUTMEG

¼ TEASPOON GROUND GINGER

PINCH GROUND CLOVES

2 CUPS ICE

1. Place the almond milk, avocado, stevia, vanilla extract, cinnamon, nutmeg, ginger, and cloves in a blender and purée until smooth.

2. Add the ice and purée until the drink is a thick milkshake texture before serving.

CALORIES: 263   TOTAL FAT: 24 G   SATURATED FAT: 4 G   SUGAR: 1 G   CARBOHYDRATES: 12 G

Refreshing Lemon-Limeade

Nothing seems to quench a raging thirst better on a hot day than a big glass of tart lemonade, so this drink will be a welcome addition to your repertoire if you live in a hot climate. There is an added benefit from enjoying this drink: Lemons are a powerful candida fighter. The antifungal properties of lemons can help detox the liver, making the organ a more effective fighter against candida.

2½ CUPS WATER

JUICE OF 2 LEMONS

JUICE OF 1 LIME

12 TO 14 DROPS LIQUID STEVIA

MINT LEAVES, FOR GARNISH

1. In a medium pitcher, stir together the water, lemon juice, lime juice, and stevia.

2. Add more stevia until the lemon-limeade suits your palate.

3. Chill the drink in the fridge and serve it over ice garnished with a few mint leaves.

CALORIES: 15   TOTAL FAT: 1 G   SATURATED FAT: 0 G   SUGAR: 1 G   CARBOHYDRATES: 1 G

Icy Vanilla Milkshake

You can use any nut milk for this creamy treat, including almond or cashew milk. You might want to make this drink as dessert, because it is as thick and satisfying as an old-fashioned drugstore milkshake. You might need a spoon instead of a straw.

2 CUPS UNSWEETENED COCONUT MILK

1 AVOCADO, PEELED, PITTED, AND HALVED

3 TEASPOONS ALCOHOL-FREE VANILLA EXTRACT

8 DROPS STEVIA

PINCH GROUND NUTMEG

2 CUPS ICE

1. Place the milk, avocado, vanilla, stevia, and nutmeg in a blender and pulse until completely smooth.

2. Add the ice and blend until the drink is a thick milkshake texture before serving.

CALORIES: 274 TOTAL FAT: 25 G SATURATED FAT: 9 G SUGAR: 1 G CARBOHYDRATES: 11 G

Simple Citrus-Spinach Cocktail

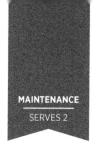

If you use field cucumbers for this drink, it is better to peel them and take the seeds out with a spoon because the skin can be tough and the seeds fibrous. Field cucumbers are typically smaller than English cucumbers, so if using that variety you can certainly add a full cucumber to this cocktail; consider it an extra dose of vitamins. Try to find English cucumbers in your local store whenever possible; they are long and slender with a lightly textured, thin skin.

3 CUPS PACKED BABY SPINACH

½ CUCUMBER

½ CUP FRESHLY SQUEEZED
    ORANGE JUICE

1 TEASPOON ORANGE ZEST

ICE CUBES

1. Place the spinach, cucumber, orange juice, and orange zest in a blender and pulse until smooth. Add more orange juice if needed.

2. Serve the cocktail over ice.

CALORIES: 51   TOTAL FAT: 1 G   SATURATED FAT: 0 G   SUGAR: 5 G   CARBOHYDRATES: 11 G

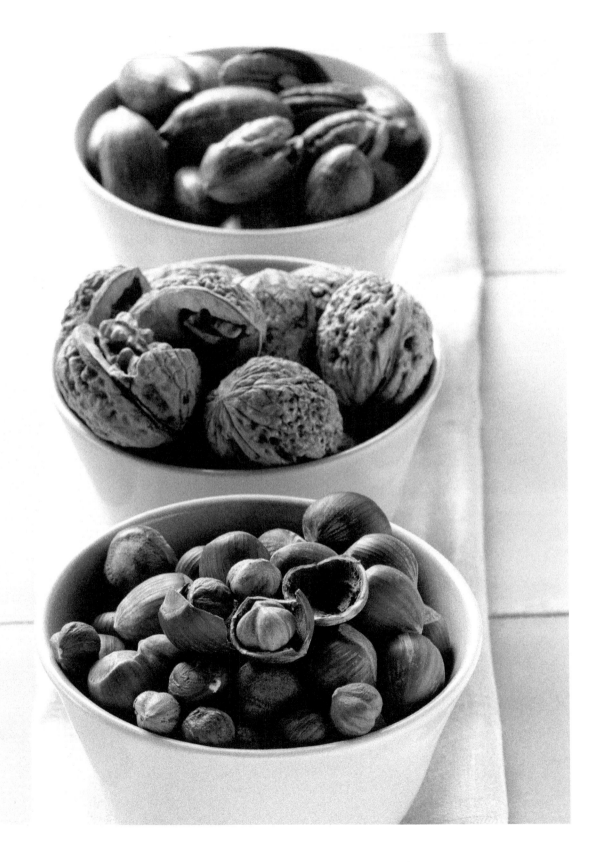

The Dirty Dozen and the Clean Fifteen

EATING CLEAN

Each year, Environmental Working Group, an environmental organization based in the United States, publishes a list they call the "Dirty Dozen." These are the fruits and vegetables that, when conventionally grown using chemical pesticides and fertilizers, carry the highest residues. If organically grown isn't an option for you, simply avoid these fruits and vegetables altogether. The list is updated each year, but here is the most recent list (2013).

Similarly, the Environmental Working Group publishes a list of "The Clean Fifteen," fruits and vegetables that, even when conventionally grown, contain very low levels of chemical pesticide or fertilizer residue. These items are acceptable to purchase conventionally grown.

You might want to snap a photo of these two lists and keep them on your phone to reference while shopping. Or you can download the Environmental Working Groups app to your phone or tablet.

THE DIRTY DOZEN

APPLE
STRAWBERRY
GRAPE
CELERY
PEACH
SPINACH
SWEET BELL
    PEPPER
IMPORTED
    NECTARINE
CUCUMBER
CHERRY TOMATO
SNAP PEA
POTATO

THE CLEAN FIFTEEN

ASPARAGUS
AVOCADO
CABBAGE
CANTALOUPE
CORN
EGGPLANT
GRAPEFRUIT
KIWI
MANGO
MUSHROOM
ONIONS
PAPAYA
PINEAPPLE
SWEET PEAS
    (FROZEN)
SWEET POTATO

Conversion Charts

VOLUME EQUIVALENTS (LIQUID)

U.S. STANDARD	U.S. STANDARD (OUNCES)	METRIC (APPROXIMATE)
2 TABLESPOONS	1 FL. OUNCE	30 MILLILITERS
¼ CUP	2 FL. OUNCES	60 MILLILITERS
½ CUP	4 FL. OUNCES	120 MILLILITERS
1 CUP	8 FL. OUNCES	240 MILLILITERS
1½ CUPS	12 FL. OUNCES	355 MILLILITERS
2 CUPS OR 1 PINT	16 FL. OUNCES	475 MILLILITERS
4 CUPS OR 1 QUART	32 FL. OUNCES	1 LITER
1 GALLON	128 FL. OUNCES	4 LITERS

OVEN TEMPERATURES

FAHRENHEIT (F)	CELSIUS (C) (APPROXIMATE)
250	120
300	150
325	165
350	180
375	190
400	200
425	220
450	230

VOLUME EQUIVALENTS (DRY)

U.S. STANDARD	METRIC (APPROXIMATE)
⅛ TEASPOON	.5 MILLILITER
¼ TEASPOON	1 MILLILITER
½ TEASPOON	2 MILLILITERS
¾ TEASPOON	4 MILLILITERS
1 TEASPOON	5 MILLILITERS
1 TABLESPOON	15 MILLILITERS
¼ CUP	59 MILLILITERS
⅓ CUP	79 MILLILITERS
½ CUP	118 MILLILITERS
⅔ CUP	156 MILLILITERS
¾ CUP	177 MILLILITERS
1 CUP	235 MILLILITERS
2 CUPS OR 1 PINT	475 MILLILITERS
3 CUPS	700 MILLILITERS
4 CUPS OR 1 QUART	1 LITER
½ GALLON	2 LITERS
1 GALLON	4 LITERS

WEIGHT EQUIVALENTS

U.S. STANDARD	METRIC (APPROXIMATE)
½ OUNCE	15 GRAMS
1 OUNCE	30 GRAMS
2 OUNCES	60 GRAMS
4 OUNCES	115 GRAMS
8 OUNCES	225 GRAMS
12 OUNCES	340 GRAMS
16 OUNCES OR 1 POUND	455 GRAMS

References

Adëeva. "The Infection-Fighting Benefits of Oregano." Accessed March 16, 2014. http://adeeva .com/documents/oregano_addl_info.pdf.

American Academy of Allergy, Asthma and Immunology (AAAAI). "Physician Reference Materials: Position Statement 14—Candidiasis Hypersensitivity Syndrome." Accessed March 15, 2014. http://web.archive.org/web/20010609033347/www.aaaai.org/professional/ physicianreference/positionstatements/ps14.stm.

Anti Candida Diet Plan. "Losing Weight While on the Candida Diet." Accessed March 15, 2014. http://anticandidadietplan.com/losing-weight-while-on-the-candida-diet/.

Bailey, Eileen. "Candida Yeast." Health Central. Accessed March 18, 2014. http://www .healthcentral.com/adhd/alternative-treatments-200132-5.html.

Bakker, Eric. "Functional Testing for Candida: The Organic Acids Urine Test." YeastInfection .org. Last modified July 13, 2013. http://www.yeastinfection.org/functional-testing-for-candida-the -organic-acids-urine-test/.

Barrett, Stephen. "Dubious 'Yeast Allergies.'" Quackwatch. Last modified October 8, 2005. http://www.quackwatch.com/01QuackeryRelatedTopics/candida.html.

Bauer, Brent A. "What Is a Candida Cleanse Diet and What Does It Do?" Mayo Clinic. September 3, 2011. http://www.mayoclinic.org/candida-cleanse/expert-answers/faq-20058174.

Bénoliel, P. "Treatment of Sino-nasal Polyposis by *Candida albicans* Immunotherapy: Apropos of 4 Cases." *Allergie et Immunologie (Paris)* 33, no. 10 (December 2001): 388–94. http://www.ncbi .nlm.nih.gov/pubmed/11802479.

Centers for Disease Control and Prevention. "Candidiasis." Last modified February 13, 2014. http://www.cdc.gov/fungal/diseases/candidiasis/index.html.

Centers for Disease Control and Prevention. "Chronic Fatigue Syndrome (CFS)." Accessed March 14, 2014. http://www.cdc.gov/cfs/causes/ and http://www.cdc.gov/cfs/.

Connealy, Leigh Erin. "The Candida and Fungus among Us." Natural News. April 23, 2008. http://www.naturalnews.com/023084_bacteria_candida_health.html#.

Crook, William. "The Effects of Candida on Mental Health." Safe Harbor. Accessed March 16, 2014. http://www.alternativementalhealth.com/articles/candida.htm.

Denver Naturopathic Clinic. "Celiac Disease, Gluten Ataxia and Candidiasis." *DNC News*. Accessed March 15, 2014. http://www.denvernaturopathic.com/news/celiac.html.

Edwards, John E., Jr. "Systemic Symptoms from Candida in the Gut: Real or Imaginary?" *Bulletin of the New York Academy of Medicine* 64, no. 6 (July-August 1988): 544–49. http://www.ncbi.nlm.nih.gov/pmc/articles/PMC1630581/.

EMedicineHealth. "Definition of *Candida albicans*." Accessed March 16, 2014. http://www.emedicinehealth.com/script/main/art.asp?articlekey=11072.

Fisher, J. F., W. H. Chew, S. Shadomy, R. J. Duma, C. G. Mayhall, and W. C. House. "Urinary Tract Infections Due to *Candida albicans*." *Review of Infectious Diseases* 4, no. 6 (November-December 1982): 1107–18. http://www.ncbi.nlm.nih.gov/pubmed/6760338.

FTC News Release. "FTC Charges Nature's Way Products' Ads for 'Cantrol' Were False and Unsubstantiated." Casewatch. August 26, 2006. http://www.casewatch.org/ftc/news/1990/cantrol.shtml.

Fushimi, T., K. Suruga, Y. Oshima, M. Fukiharu, Y. Tsukamoto, and T. Goda. "Dietary Acetic Acid Reduces Serum Cholesterol and Triacylglycerols in Rats Fed a Cholesterol-Rich Diet." *British Journal of Nutrition* 95, no. 5 (May 2006): 916–24. http://www.ncbi.nlm.nih.gov/pubmed/16611381.

Griffin, R. Morgan. "Clearing Away MS Brain Fog." *Multiple Sclerosis Health Center*, WebMD. Accessed March 11, 2014. http://www.webmd.com/multiple-sclerosis/features/clearing_away_ms_brain_fog.

Guarner, F., and J. R. Malagelada. "Gut Flora in Health and Disease." *Lancet* 361 (February 2003): 512–19. http://www.ncbi.nlm.nih.gov/pubmed/12583961.

Guo, Ty. "*Candida albicans*, Flora and Pathogen." Biology Online. Last modified April 20, 2009. http://www.biology-online.org/biology-forum/about2921.html.

Harklute, Aurora. "How Long to Stay on Candida Diet?" LiveStrong.com. Last modified August 16, 2013. http://www.livestrong.com/article/279240-how-long-to-stay-on-candida-diet/.

Harvard Health Publications. "Benefit of Probiotics: Should You Take a Daily Dose of Bacteria?" Harvard Medical School. May 2005. http://www.health.harvard.edu/press_releases/Benefit_of_Probiotics_Should_you_take_a_daily_dose_of_bacteria.

Harvard School of Public Health Nutrition Source. "Carbohydrates and Blood Sugar." Accessed March 16, 2014. http://www.hsph.harvard.edu/nutritionsource/carbohydrates/carbohydrates-and -blood-sugar/.

Hsieh, M. H., P. Chan, Y. M. Sue, J. C. Liu, T. H. Liang, T. Y. Huang, B. Tomlinson, M. S. Chow, P. F. Kao, and Y. J. Chen. "Efficacy and Tolerability of Oral Stevioside in Patients with Mild Essential Hypertension: A Two-Year, Randomized, Placebo-Controlled Study." *Clinical Therapy* 25, no. 11 (November 2003): 2797–808. http://www.ncbi.nlm.nih.gov/pubmed/14693305.

Institute of Medicine of the National Academies. "Dietary Reference Intakes: Water, Potassium, Sodium, Chloride, and Sulfate." February 11, 2004. http://www.iom.edu/Reports/2004 /Dietary-Reference-Intakes-Water-Potassium-Sodium-Chloride-and-Sulfate.aspx.

Jagyasi, Prem. "How to Deal with Sugar Cravings." DrPrem.com. Accessed March 15, 2014. http://drprem.com/howto/sugar-cravings.html.

James, William D., Timothy Berger, and Dirk Elston. *Andrews' Diseases of the Skin: Clinical Dermatology—Expert Consult* 11th ed. New York: Saunders Elsevier, 2011.

Lucas, Cara. "Taming Candida." Alternative Medicine. Accessed March 16, 2014. http://www .alternativemedicine.com/candida/taming-candida.

Marchaim, D., L. Lemanek, S. Bheemreddy, K. S. Kaye, and J. D. Sobel. "Fluconazole-Resistant *Candida albicans* Vulvovaginitis." *Obstetrics and Gynecology* 120, no. 6 (December 2012): 1407–14. http://www.ncbi.nlm.nih.gov/pubmed/23168767.

Mathur, S., R. S. Mathur, H. Dowda, H. O. Williamson, W. P. Faulk, and H. H. Fudenberg. "Sex Steroid Hormones and Antibodies to *Candida albicans*." *Clinical and Experimental Immunology* 33, no. 1 (July 1978): 79–87. http://www.ncbi.nlm.nih.gov/pmc/articles/PMC1537510/.

McCormick, Kathleen. "Digesting It All!" *Connections*. April 2012. http://www .womensinternational.com/connections/digesting.html.

MedicineNet.com. "How Does Alcohol Affect Your Blood Sugar?" Alcohol and Nutrition. Accessed March 18, 2014. http://www.medicinenet.com/alcohol_and_nutrition/page4.htm.

Miami College of Arts and Sciences. "The Digestive System." Accessed March 13, 2014. http:// www.as.miami.edu/chemistry/2086/chap%2024/chapter%2024-newpart1.htm.

National Digestive Diseases Information Clearinghouse. "The Digestive System and How It Works." National Institute of Diabetes and Digestive and Kidney Diseases. Last modified September 18, 2013. http://digestive.niddk.nih.gov/ddiseases/pubs/yrdd/.

National Institute of Mental Health. "What Is Depression?" Accessed March 11, 2014. http://www.nimh.nih.gov/health/topics/depression/index.shtml?utm_source=BrainLine.org&utm_medium=Twitter.

National Institutes of Health. "Vaginal Yeast Infection." MedlinePlus. Last modified November 7, 2011. http://www.nlm.nih.gov/medlineplus/ency/article/001511.htm.

National Resource Center on ADHD. "Complementary and Alternative Treatments." Last modified January 2008. http://www.help4adhd.org/treatment/complementary/WWK6.

Nature. "Immunology: Controlling Natural Killers." 483 (March 2012): 249. doi:10.1038/483249b.

New York Times Staff. "Thrush." *New York Times* Health Guide. Accessed March 11, 2014. http://www.nytimes.com/health/guides/disease/thrush/overview.html.

Nordqvist, Christian. "What Is Inflammation? What Causes Inflammation?" Medical News Today. July 31, 2012. http://www.medicalnewstoday.com/articles/248423.php.

Rex, J. H., M. G. Rinaldi, and M. A. Pfaller. "Resistance of Candida Species to Fluconazole." *Antimicrobial Agents and Chemotherapy* 39, no. 1 (January 1995): 1–8. http://aac.asm.org/content/39/1/1.full.pdf+html.

Rimawi, Bassam H., and Ramzy H. Rimawi. "Gynecological Infections in Immunocompromised Hosts." OMICS Group eBooks. Accessed March 13, 2014. http://www.esciencecentral.org/ebooks/bacterial-mycotic-infections/gynecological-infections.php.

Rosenbach, Ari, Daniel Dignard, Jessica V. Pierce, Malcolm Whiteway, and Carol A. Kumamoto. "Adaptations of *Candida albicans* for Growth in the Mammalian Intestinal Tract." *Eukaryotic Cell* 9, no. 7 (July 2010): 1075–86. http://www.ncbi.nlm.nih.gov/pmc/articles/PMC2901676/.

Sanglard, D., K. Kuchler, F. Ischer, J. L. Pagani, M. Monod, and J. Bille. "Mechanisms of Resistance to Azole Antifungal Agents in *Candida albicans* Isolates from AIDS Patients Involve Specific Multidrug Transporters." *Antimicrobial Agents and Chemotherapy* 39, no. 11 (November 1995): 2378–86. http://www.ncbi.nlm.nih.gov/pubmed/8585712.

Science*Daily.* "Microflora Have Decisive Role with Autoimmune Illnesses, Some Good, Some Bad." April 5, 2012. http://www.sciencedaily.com/releases/2012/04/120405075223.htm.

Sims, C. R., L. Ostrosky-Zeichner, and J. H. Rex. "Invasive Candidiasis in Immunocompromised Hospitalized Patients." *Archives of Medical Research* 36, no. 6 (November-December 2005): 660–71. http://www.ncbi.nlm.nih.gov/pubmed/16216647.

Smart Nutrition. "Candida Albicans." Accessed March 18, 2014. http://www.smartnutrition
.co.uk/ibs-gut-disorder-clinics/digestive-health/candida-albicans/.

Snyder Sachs, Jessica. "Best Cure for Stomach Troubles—Which Probiotics Work and Why."
Health Magazine. Last modified March 10, 2009. http://www.cnn.com/2009/HEALTH/03/10
/healthmag.probiotics.stomach/index.html?eref=rss_latest.

Sobel, Jack D. "Patient Information: Vaginal Yeast Infection (Beyond the Basics)." UpToDate.
Last modified December 10, 2013. http://www.uptodate.com/contents/vaginal-yeast-infection
-beyond-the-basics.

TheCandidaDiet.com. "Antifungals: Caprylic Acid." Accessed March 18, 2014. http://www
.thecandidadiet.com/caprylicacid.htm.

TheCandidaDiet.com. "Candida Die-Off: Symptoms and Treatment. Accessed March 18, 2014.
http://www.thecandidadiet.com/candida-die-off.htm.

TheCandidaDiet.com. "Your Candida Cleanse." Accessed March 18, 2014. http://www
.thecandidadiet.com/cleansing.htm.

Total Health Institute. "Autoimmune and Allergy." Accessed March 18, 2014. http://www
.totalhealthinstitute.com/autoimmune-and-allergy/.

U.S. Food and Drug Administration (FDA). "GRAS Notice (GRN) No. 449." Accessed March 20,
2014. http://www.accessdata.fda.gov/scripts/fdcc/?set=GRASNotices.

U.S. Food and Drug Administration (FDA). "What Refined Stevia Preparations Have Been
Evaluated by FDA to Be Used As a Sweetener?" Last modified April 4, 2012. http://www.fda.gov
/aboutfda/transparency/basics/ucm214865.htm.

Vargas, S. L., C. C. Patrick, G. D. Ayers, and W. T. Hughes. "Modulating Effect of Dietary
Carbohydrate Supplementation on *Candida albicans* Colonization and Invasion in a Neutropenic
Mouse Model." *Infection and Immunology* 61, no. 2 (February 1993): 619–26. http://www.ncbi.nlm
.nih.gov/pubmed/8423091.

WebMD. "Apple Cider Vinegar." Accessed March 24, 2014. http://www.webmd.com/diet
/apple-cider-vinegar?page=2.

WebMD. "Drugs and Medications—Fluconazole Oral." Accessed March 18, 2014.
http://www.webmd.com/drugs/mono-5052-FLUCONAZOLE+-.+ORAL
.aspx?drugid=3780&drugname=fluconazole+oral&source=0&pagenumber=4.

Weig, Michael, Edgar Werner, Matthias Frosch, and Heinrich Kasper. "Limited Effect of Refined Carbohydrate Dietary Supplementation on Colonization of the Gastrointestinal Tract of Healthy Subjects by *Candida albicans.*" *American Journal of Clinical Nutrition* 69, no. 6 (June 1999): 1170–73. http://www.ncbi.nlm.nih.gov/pubmed/10357735.

White, Andrea M., and Carol S. Johnston. "Vinegar Ingestion at Bedtime Moderates Waking Glucose Concentrations in Adults with Well-Controlled Type 2 Diabetes." *Diabetes Care* 30, no. 11 (November 2007): 2814–15. http://care.diabetesjournals.org/content/30/11/2814.full.

WholeApproach. "Diagnosing Candida." Accessed March 16, 2014. http://www.wholeapproach.com/candida/diagnosingcandida.php.

Williams, David. "Which Probiotic Bacteria Have the Most Digestive Benefits." *Dr. David Williams* (blog). Accessed March 13, 2014. http://www.drdavidwilliams.com/digestive-health-probiotic-strains/#axzz2sUk26Max.

Yeast Connection, The. Accessed March 13, 2014. http://www.yeastconnection.com.

Zwolińska-Wcisło, M., A. Budak, D. Tojanowska, T. Mach, L. Rudnicka-Sosin, D. Galicka-Latała, P. Nowak, and D. Cibor. (Jagiellonian University, Poland.) "The Influence of *Candida albicans* on the Course of Ulcerative Colitis." *Przegląd Lekarski* 63, no. 7 (2006): 533–38. http://www.ncbi.nlm.nih.gov/pubmed/17203803.

Recipe Index

Index

Lightning Source UK Ltd.
Milton Keynes UK
UKOW07f0331110417
298855UK00003B/5/P